anti-inflammatory
FOODS AND RECIPES

USING THE POWER OF PLANT FOODS TO HEAL AND PREVENT
arthritis, cancer, diabetes, heart disease, and chronic pain

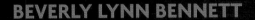

BEVERLY LYNN BENNETT

Book Publishing Company
SUMMERTOWN, TENNESSEE

Library of Congress Cataloging-in-Publication Data

Names: Bennett, Beverly Lynn, author.
Title: Anti-inflammatory foods and recipes : using the power of plant foods
    to heal and prevent arthritis, cancer, diabetes, heart disease, and
    chronic pain / Beverly Lynn Bennett.
Description: Summertown, Tennessee : Book Publishing Company, [2017] |
    Includes index.
Identifiers: LCCN 2017007125 | ISBN 9781570673412 (pbk.)
Subjects: LCSH: Inflammation—Diet therapy. | Inflammation—Diet
    therapy—Recipes.
Classification: LCC RB131 .B46 2017 | DDC 616/.0473—dc23
LC record available at https://lccn.loc.gov/2017007125

Nutrition Breakdowns for Recipes: The nutrient values provided for the recipes in this book are estimates only, calculated from the individual ingredients used in each recipe based on the nutrition data found for those ingredients. Optional items are not included. Nutrient content may vary based on methods of preparation, origin and freshness of ingredients, product brands, and other factors.

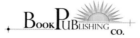

We chose to print this title on responsibly harvested paper stock certified by The Forest Stewardship Council, an independent auditor of responsible forestry practices. For more information, visit us.fsc.org.

Cover and interior design: John Wincek
Food styling and photography: Alan Roettinger
Stock photography: 123 RF

Printed in Canada

Book Publishing Company
PO Box 99
Summertown, TN 38483
888-260-8458
bookpubco.com

ISBN: 978-1-57067-341-2

22 21 20 19 18 17   1 2 3 4 5 6 7 8 9

Disclaimer: The information in this book is presented for educational purposes only. It isn't intended to be a substitute for the medical advice of a physician, dietitian, or other healthcare professional.

contents

CHAPTER 1 defining inflammation 1

CHAPTER 2 what is chronic inflammation? 7

CHAPTER 3 how to fight chronic inflammation 17

CHAPTER 4 anti-inflammatory foods, nutrients, and supplements 25

CHAPTER 5 beverages and breakfast 33

CHAPTER 6 fermented foods, sauces, and spreads 47

CHAPTER 7 slaws and salads 53

CHAPTER 8 soups and stews 63

CHAPTER 9 side dishes 74

CHAPTER 10 main dishes 93

CHAPTER 11 sweet treats 103

index *116*

anti-inflammatory
FOODS AND RECIPES

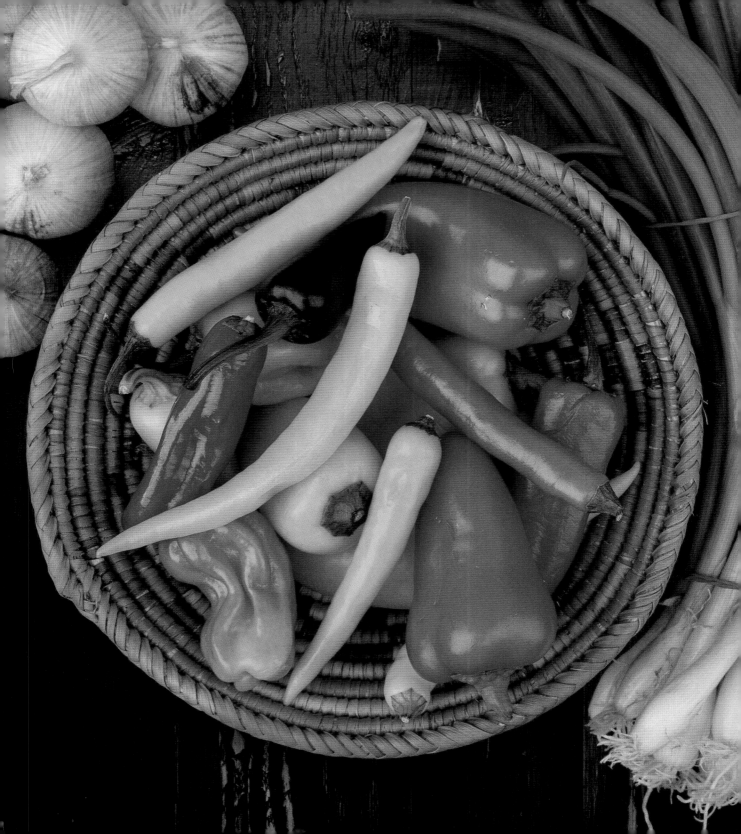

defining inflammation

Inflammation is either the cause or consequence of nearly every injury, infection, and disease, and sometimes it's both. In a nutshell, inflammation is the immune system's defense mechanism in action. Under normal circumstances, inflammation occurs in response to an injury or infection and then stops once the problem has resolved. This is called acute, or useful, inflammation, and its symptoms are unmistakable. The root of the word "inflammation" derives from the Latin *inflammare*, which means "to catch fire" or "to burst into flames." This term encompasses the four symptoms that arise when the body experiences inflammation: redness, heat, swelling, and pain.

After an injury—whether it's a sprained wrist, a stubbed toe, a pinched finger, or an insect bite—all four symptoms will appear. Redness and heat indicate that blood is flowing to the location of the injury. Swelling occurs as plasma begins to fill the surrounding tissues. Pain is the telltale sign that something is amiss—a message the body is under attack and requires immediate attention. These symptoms are often acute at first but gradually dissipate as the healing process progresses. Eventually the body returns to normal, and in most cases not even a scar remains.

Acute systemic infections (those that occur throughout the body) often take longer to manifest, but they elicit the same response from the immune system. With infection from a flu virus, for example, there might initially be a vague feeling of discomfort, followed by a burning in the eye sockets or joints, chills, and finally a fever. These are signs the body is fighting off the infection. Some people take anti-inflammatory drugs, such as ibuprofen, to relieve the discomfort. Others simply allow the fever to run its course and destroy the invading pathogen.

Allergies also trigger an inflammatory response. For instance, when people are exposed to environmental substances or foods they're allergic to, the immune system will launch an attack, causing symptoms such as a runny nose, itchy skin, or swollen joints. Usually these symptoms subside naturally once the offending allergen is removed. However, hypersensitive allergic reactions, known as anaphylaxis, can be life threatening and require immediate medical intervention.

Of course, more serious illnesses require more robust therapies. But in all cases, inflammation is the body's natural response to an invasive attack, and it usually abates once the healing is complete. Although the expression of acute inflammation can be unpleasant, it's evidence of a healthy immune system.

WHAT HAPPENS DURING INFLAMMATION

When the body needs to respond to an injury, it mobilizes an army of specialized cells and chemicals to fight invading organisms and toxins. The specialized cells prepare pathways for fighter cells to attack and engulf the unwelcome invaders. Next, another group of cells signals the body that the fighter cells have been successful, which stops the production of the preparatory and fighter cells and triggers the appearance of cleanup and repair cells to clear the battlefield of debris and mend any damage.

Simply put, there are two stages to the inflammatory response: pro-inflammatory and anti-inflammatory. Each participating cell in the pro-inflammatory stage builds on the work of the previous cells and makes the immune reaction stronger. During the pro-inflammatory period, symptoms such as pain, itching, redness, heat, or swelling arise. The anti-inflammatory process puts out the fire, reversing the pro-inflammatory reaction and returning the body to normal.

A number of substances that either cause or block inflammation are made from essential fatty acids, which are fats the body cannot produce on its own. These fatty acids must be obtained from foods or supplements. There are two families of essential fats: omega-3s and omega-6s. Omega-6 fatty acids tend to increase inflammation; omega-3 fatty acids help to curtail it. It's important to remember that in a more complex depiction of the process of inflammation, some of these substances have multiple roles, including promoting the battle phase of inflammation and subsequently shutting it down when it's no longer necessary. The most common roles are explained in the descriptions that follow.

The Preparatory Substances

A number of different substances work together to alert the body there's been an injury. Other substances prepare the area around the injury to make it easier for healing substances to fight harmful invading microbes.

Histamine. White blood cells near the injury site release a substance called histamine, which increases the permeability of blood vessels around a wound. This signals fighter cells and other substances that regulate the immune response to come to the site of the injury. They gain easier access to the site because histamine makes the surrounding blood vessels more porous. Histamine also instigates swelling and redness around the site of the injury. Its effects are particularly noticeable during an allergic reaction, when symptoms might include a runny nose, itchy eyes, or a rash.

Eicosanoids. Eicosanoids are signaling molecules produced from essential fatty acids. They can be either pro-inflammatory or anti-inflammatory depending on which family of essential fats they come from. Pro-inflammatory eicosanoids continue the work of histamines, increasing the permeability of blood vessels, which causes the swelling associated with inflammation. Prostaglandins are one of the primary pro-inflammatory eicosanoids; they make blood vessels more porous, create heat or fever to kill invading pathogens, and induce pain, which helps immobilize the injured area. Leukotrienes are another primary pro-inflammatory eicosanoid, and they also make blood vessels more porous and send signals to fighter cells to help them locate the injury. In addition, leukotrienes restrict airways and create nasal mucus, in much the same way that histamine does but more intensely. Pain is caused initially by the swelling that activates the immediate nerve endings adjacent to an injury. Pro-inflammatory eicosanoids increase the sensitivity of these nerves.

Cytokines. Cytokines are proteins activated by pro-inflammatory eicosanoids to signal fighter cells to gather at the injury site. In addition, they're responsible for diverting energy to the healing process. As a result, the release of cytokines may cause tiredness and decreased appetite because the digestive process requires a certain amount of energy and also supplies the body with energy. It's thought that the reason so many relatively healthy people died during the Spanish flu outbreak of 1918 was because that particular viral strain stimulated unusually strong immune reactions. Healthy individuals produced such high levels of cytokines in response to the virus that their bodies couldn't regulate the ensuing inflammation.

C-reactive protein. Cytokines, along with other pro-inflammatory eicosanoids, are involved in the activation of a substance called C-reactive protein (CRP). This is an organic compound produced by the liver that responds to messages sent out by white blood cells in response to infection. C-reactive proteins bind to the site of the injury and act like the surveillance team in a battle, identifying which substances are foreign to the body.

Many of the participating substances in the immune response are only present for a short time—just a few seconds in some cases. C-reactive protein is an exception. Because it remains at measurable levels for up to two days, researchers and physicians often use it to gauge how much inflammation is present in the body.

The Active Fighters

Once the preparatory substances have readied a wound site, active fighters come into play. These microorganisms are responsible for destroying pathogens.

Leukocytes (neutrophils and macrophages). Several types of leukocytes, also known as white blood cells, are critical to the process of neutralizing invading substances. Neutrophils, which are small and agile, are the first to arrive at the scene of an injury to engulf and ingest microbes. However, neutrophils aren't able to digest all types of pathogens, so they're aided by macrophages, another type of leukocyte. Macrophages are larger than neutrophils and can tackle greater numbers of invading organisms. They have a longer life cycle than neutrophils, and certain macrophages also help with the repair process.

Free radicals. Both neutrophils and macrophages are coated with highly reactive substances called free radicals that kill invading pathogens. Free radicals are unstable molecules that trigger chemical reactions more readily than stable substances. Through a series of reactions, some of the free radicals on the surfaces of these leukocytes turn into hydrogen peroxide, and some of this hydrogen peroxide is then converted into hypochlorite—better known as chlorine bleach. Anyone who's familiar with these two substances will recognize them as lethal, not only to unwanted invaders but also to healthy cells as well. If there's any upset in the finely tuned balance of the immune system, which regulates inflammation and the production of these substances, there could be a resultant cascade of damage and disease.

Leukocytes are protected from the harmful chemicals that surround them because they contain large amounts of antioxidants, which are substances that neutralize free radicals. If the supply of antioxidants drops too low, leukocytes will become endangered and won't be able to fight off infection. However, if antioxidant stores become too high, the free radicals needed to fight infection will be compromised. In order for the immune system to function optimally and successfully, the many substances it relies on must maintain a delicate balance.

REVERSING THE INFLAMMATION PROCESS

Once the invading pathogens have been neutralized, inflammation subsides and the healing phase begins. According to medical researcher and biochemist Barry Sears, author of *The Anti-Inflammation Zone*, the overall inflammation process can be broken down into four stages: recall, resolution, regeneration, and repair.

Macrophages not only ingest invading organisms, but they also clean up the debris that remains after the battle, including any neutrophils that are no longer viable. There are several other substances that also play a role in resolving inflammation and repairing the injured area:

Cortisol. The adrenal glands produce cortisol, a steroid that turns off the activity of a number of the cells that prepare the body to fight infection.

Resolvins. Resolvins are part of a group of specialized compounds derived from eicosanoids, most of which are formed from omega-3 fatty acids, that tamp down the inflammatory response. Resolvins reduce the number of white blood cells circulating near the injured area and help encourage macrophages to clean up cell debris and toxins.

Protectins. Protectins are also formed from omega-3 fatty acids and are important for halting the production of prostaglandins and stopping cell degeneration. They are particularly active in the lungs and brain.

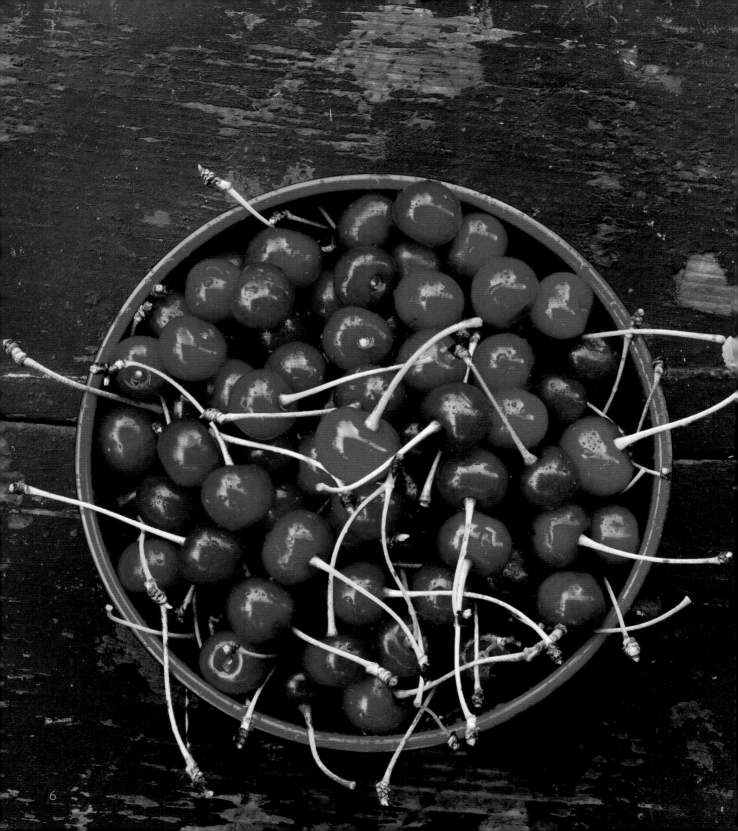

what is chronic inflammation?

Acute inflammation damages both good and bad cells alike, so the body keeps a tight check on it. However, for reasons not yet well understood, certain triggers can disrupt the fine balance that regulates the inflammatory process, resulting in chronic, or ongoing, inflammation. For example, when cortisol is released in just the right amount and for just the right length of time to stop the inflammatory process, this is a useful response. However, when cortisol is released, it circulates throughout the body, not just at the site of injury, and if it travels systemically on a regular basis, it ends up hindering the immune system overall. Not only will the continued presence of cortisol slow healing, but it will also heighten insulin resistance, leading to weight gain and negatively affecting brain cells that control memory. In general, chronic inflammation is particularly bad for the heart and brain because the cells of these organs are very slow to regenerate when damaged—if they regenerate at all.

AILMENTS CAUSED BY CHRONIC INFLAMMATION

 hronic, silent, or unproductive inflammation may be present in the body for years with no obvious symptoms. Think of it as a slow burn that goes unnoticed until considerable damage is done. Chronic inflammation follows the same process as acute inflammation, except it initially operates below the pain threshold and isn't temporary. If left unchecked, chronic inflammation can lead to serious health problems.

Cancer. Cancerous tumors secrete substances that attract cytokines (see page 3) and free radicals (see page 4), cells that cause inflammation, and use them to help the tumor survive. These substances also help loose tumor cells attach to new sites so they can grow and spread. When the body is already fighting inflammation from other causes, it can become fertile ground for cancer cell activity.

Diabetes. High insulin levels increase the activity of a substance called enzyme D5D, which increases production of the inflammatory omega-6 fat arachidonic acid. Consequently, inflammation can compromise the activity of the endothelial cells that line blood vessels, making it difficult for insulin to access other cells and help them take in glucose, which in turn causes insulin levels in the bloodstream to rise. Inflammation then creates a link between diabetes and heart disease: insulin activates D5D, which creates more inflammatory arachidonic acid and blood vessel damage.

Heart disease. Pro-inflammatory eicosanoids, such as arachidonic acid, can cause a plaque inside an artery to rupture, attracting platelets that could form blood clots and aggregate to create a blockage. They also could cause an artery to spasm. Inadequate levels of omega-3 fatty acids can lead to an irregular heartbeat, which contributes to heart attacks.

Alzheimer's disease. The brain doesn't have any pain receptors, so we can't feel the effects that chronic inflammation has on it. Researchers have found that people with high levels of omega-6 fatty acids have a much greater incidence of Alzheimer's disease. In particular, the Framingham Heart Study showed that people with the lowest levels of circulating omega-3s had the highest rates of Alzheimer's disease, although researchers don't fully understand why. There is also speculation about the connection between Alzheimer's disease and diabetes; factors involved in insulin resistance also promote plaque development in the brain.

In some cases the immune response will turn against the body itself. Autoimmune diseases, such as lupus, rheumatoid arthritis, and type 1 diabetes, are actually forms of chronic inflammation. Common symptoms of autoimmune diseases are allergies, asthma, chronic fatigue, joint pain, skin problems (including eczema, premature aging, and wrinkling), and even depression. Allergies are a form of immune response to various substances that most people's bodies would treat as harmless.

Chronic inflammation also contributes to and accelerates the aging process by prohibiting cell growth and regeneration. A 2014 study conducted at the University of Bologna that was published in *The Journals of Gerontology* showed how chronic, low-grade inflammation is inevitable during the process of aging. This relationship, called inflammaging, isn't yet well understood, but scientists do know that the greater the measureable inflammatory response in an elderly person, the greater the risk of illness and death. Gerontologists specializing in this area of research are currently exploring this association and testing promising treatments that might help reduce inflammaging.

One possible cause of inflammaging is the amount of cell debris that accumulates as people get older. The body responds to cell debris as if it were a foreign substance, which in healthy individuals triggers macrophages that engulf and dispose of it. As we age, the disposal process becomes less effective, but the continued presence of debris causes the body to maintain an inflammatory response in an attempt to remove these unwelcome substances. Another potential cause is the action of the gut flora residing in the large intestine. During the aging process, the large intestine becomes more permeable and less able to keep these mostly beneficial organisms from moving out of the intestine and into the body; this migration may trigger inflammaging. It's also conceivable the organisms themselves might change in ways that cause inflammation.

Healthy cells are coded to prevent them from growing out of control, as happens with cancer. As cells age, this coding becomes persistent and prevents cell growth from occurring when it would be beneficial. Preventing unwanted cell growth is part of the inflammatory response, so cells that persistently shut down growth also trigger additional inflammation. Interestingly, cells that are signaling to slow growth are found in especially high levels in body fat, suggesting a link between obesity and inflammaging.

With age, blood coagulation capacity increases, which is also a part of the inflammatory response. This tendency may be responsible for the increased risk of dangerous blood clots in elderly individuals. The immune system may also experience the burden of a lifetime of toxic exposure, and parts of that system may decline while other parts become more active, contributing to inflammation. An immune system that is defective or functioning improperly could also lead to macular degeneration, one the principal drivers of blindness in older people.

People who live exceptionally long lives, especially those who do so in good health, offer an interesting counterpoint to the observation that chronic inflammation and aging are inevitably linked. The researchers involved with the University of Bologna study speculate that the usual methods for measuring inflammation might not be as accurate for predicting the potential for illness as was once thought. A small amount of chronic inflammation may always be present in the body, not as a response to illness or injury but as a normal part of cell death and regeneration. Also, some lucky individuals may have a genetic ability to create more of an anti-inflammatory response than other people do. As a result, they might experience less inflammaging in their later years.

THE CAUSES OF CHRONIC INFLAMMATION

Chronic inflammation is most commonly caused by exposure to toxins and poor lifestyle choices. As noted previously, it can also be a natural component of the aging process.

Lifestyle Factors

Fortunately, many causes of chronic inflammation are linked to harmful habits that are within our control. By understanding how these factors influence inflammation, we can make positive lifestyle changes to improve our health.

Diet

More causes of inflammation are related to diet than any other factor. Top on the list of harmful substances are refined fats, refined carbohydrates, and animal products.

Although carbohydrates and fats don't contribute directly to inflammation, refined foods deliver a higher concentration of carbs and fats than is found naturally in foods. It's thought that these higher concentrations adversely affect gut flora in ways that increase inflammatory factors. When the body is in the throes of chronic inflammation, refined foods will have an even greater negative impact on gut flora.

The types of fats a person consumes can affect inflammation in a variety of ways. Before the advent of processed foods, the human diet had a nearly equal balance of omega-3 and omega-6 fats. Most modern diets contain much higher amounts of omega-6 fats as opposed to omega-3s, and in some cases, ten to twenty times as much. It's important to ensure an adequate supply of omega-3 fatty acids because omega-6s and omega-3s compete for the same COX enzymes, which are enzymes needed to build larger fat molecules. COX-2 enzymes in particular are essential for making inflammatory prostaglandins. If too many omega-6 fats are consumed, they'll dominate the use of these enzymes, decreasing the body's ability to build anti-inflammatory fats from omega-3s.

Fats that have been chemically modified can also contribute to inflammation. Early in the twentieth century, manufacturers sought inexpensive alternatives to solid fats. Because liquid oils were cheap and plentiful, food chemists explored ways to alter the composition of these oils to create solids. Their resulting discovery was what's now known as trans fats, which manufacturers used to make vegetable shortening and margarine. Unfortunately, no one realized at the time that the unnatural chemical structure of trans fats causes them to disrupt the normal flow of nutrients in and out of cell membranes and also allows harmful substances to enter cells. In addition, trans fats interfere with the action of COX-2 enzymes, resulting in the production of cytokines that signal the need for inflammation to begin, along with the release of C-reactive protein to assist the healing process.

Fats are also chemically modified when they're subjected to very high heat. When foods are fried, for example, toxic substances called advanced glycation end products (AGES) are created from both fats and proteins. After these foods are ingested, immune cells produce large amounts of cytokines in an attempt to protect the body from these harmful substances.

Animal products—especially meat and dairy products—contain higher amounts of pro-inflammatory essential fats, such as arachidonic acid, than whole plant foods. In addition, these animal-derived items introduce more pathogenic microbes into the body, triggering an immune response. Even when these foods are cooked at high temperatures or their pH is greatly acidified (such as by marinating them in lemon juice or vinegar), the toxins produced by the microbes they contain still exert an inflammatory load on the body. Also, red meat contains a type of simple sugar called N-glycolylneuraminic acid (Neu5Gc) that the human body is unable to process because it lacks the necessary enzyme. All other meat-eating animals carry this enzyme. Consumption of foods containing Neu5Ge creates an immune response in humans that is linked to certain cancers.

Aging

The natural aging process creates inflammation and is also a result of it. As we age, fewer cells regenerate as they die, leaving behind more cell debris to trigger inflammation. Cells that don't regenerate properly or adequately increase the presence of the inflammatory substances needed to remove damaged proteins. As we age, mitochondria (the parts of cells responsible for energy production) perform less effectively and become unable to properly regulate cell death. This causes some cells to die prematurely and others to perform inefficiently, both of which could trigger an immune response. As immune-fighting cells age, they have a more difficult time recognizing harmful microorganisms that need to be removed. The adrenal hormone dehydroepiandrosterone (DHEA) and sex hormones are useful in suppressing cytokines when needed, but the production of each of these regulatory substances declines with age.

Hormone Replacement Therapy

Researchers at the University of Alabama found that oral estrogen can increase C-reactive protein (CRP) levels but that transdermal estrogen (estrogen that's applied to the skin) does not. Although elevated CRP levels are associated with greater risk of heart disease, it's not yet clear whether the rise in CRP associated with oral hormone therapy actually increases vascular disease.

Obesity, Inactivity, and Exercise

Inactivity can lead to obesity, which itself can cause inflammation. Adipose tissue, the layer of fat found beneath the skin, does much more than insulate the body. It's also metabolically active, which means it causes changes to the body's chemistry and is also changed by various body systems. This fat contains many white blood cells, so the greater the amount of body fat, the greater the number of white blood cells present. These cells release pro-inflammatory substances, especially those that promote insulin resistance.

Exercise and activity release myokines, a type of cytokine, from adipose fat and muscle tissue. Myokines stop the action of pro-inflammatory substances. Their action is particularly important for reducing the effects of insulin resistance.

Sleep Deprivation

Researchers know that a lack of sleep is associated with illness, but they don't yet understand why. So far, studies show that when we don't get enough sleep, certain infection-fighting white blood cells, known as T-cells, decrease, and the number of inflammation-promoting cytokines goes up.

Stress

Cortisol is a hormone produced by the adrenal glands to manage the body's response to stress. It stimulates a burst of energy and suppresses the action of pro-inflammatory substances. Cortisol reduces stress in the short term by counteracting pro-inflammatory eicosanoids and depleting DHEA. But too much cortisol causes immune cells to lose their sensitivity to the hormone, eventually triggering inflammation.

Sun Exposure

It was once commonly thought that individuals with dark skin have a much lower risk of health problems related to excessive sun exposure than those who are fair. However, studies have shown that both dark-skinned and light-skinned people experience reduced immune responses when overexposed to sunlight. Too much exposure, enough to cause sunburn, creates free radicals below the skin's surface. Free radicals (see page 4) are unstable molecules that destroy injury-fighting cells and reduce the number of white blood cells that fight damaging microbes. For instance, when the lips are exposed to too much sun, a dormant case of herpes simplex virus can become active as a result of weakened immunity.

Exposure to Toxins

Toxins that cause inflammation can range from dangerous substances in the environment to medications. Some pharmaceuticals are extremely helpful when taken only occasionally and in small doses, but regular use of certain medications puts an unwanted load on the body's immune system.

NSAIDs

Many people commonly use nonsteroidal anti-inflammatory drugs (NSAIDs), such as aspirin, ibuprofen, and naproxen, to reduce inflammation and relieve fever and pain. While NSAIDs often do a good job of decreasing inflammation, they can come with undesirable side effects. For instance, the combination of intense exercise and NSAID use can stimulate or exacerbate leaky gut syndrome, a condition in which the small intestine becomes more permeable and allows tiny particles to penetrate the intestinal lining and travel into the bloodstream. The immune system responds to these particles as if they're foreign substances, triggering the inflammatory response.

Dutch researchers noticed that athletes often suffer from abdominal distress and cramping during competition, and the researchers decided to investigate whether NSAIDs would increase or decrease this stress. They discovered that when NSAIDs are used before or after intense exercise, there is a much higher occurrence of intestinal permeability than would be experienced with either exercise or NSAID use alone. These findings should serve as a caution to anyone who regularly takes NSAIDs to prevent soreness after a strenuous workout.

Smoking

Cigarette smoke, whether firsthand or secondhand, is one of the most health-damaging environmental toxins. When tobacco smoke is inhaled, highly reactive substances are created in the body, similar to what the immune system uses to kill invading organisms. However, these substances turn against healthy cells instead of harmful microbes, especially the cells that line the airways and lungs.

Cigarette smoke is particularly effective at crippling the body's ability to fight disease. It suppresses the capacity of white blood cells to produce substances needed for inflammatory healing. When smokers contract pneumonia, they usually become sicker and have more severe symptoms than nonsmokers. Smokers are also more likely to develop tuberculosis.

IDENTIFYING CHRONIC INFLAMMATION

Even if you appear to be in good health, you can suffer from "silent" chronic inflammation that hasn't yet manifested as discomfort or illness. That's why physicians often include tests that measure chronic inflammation as part of their routine physical exams. Most inflammatory mediators (substances that help regulate inflammation) deteriorate too quickly to be accurately measured except for C-reactive protein (CRP), fibrinogen (a soluble protein in blood plasma that helps form red blood cells), and white blood cells. The test for CRP and white blood cells involves collecting a blood sample; the results are often available in just one day. However, what's considered a "normal" level can vary from lab to lab.

Be sure to tell your health provider if you've recently been injured, had surgery, or undergone strenuous exercise. These factors can temporarily raise markers for inflammation and cause inaccurate test results, so it might be good to delay the test for a few days until your body recovers or normalizes.

Barry Sears, a pioneer in biotechnology specializing in the impact of diet on inflammation, is a proponent of testing the levels of two essential fatty acids in the blood: arachidonic acid (an omega-6 fat) and eicosapentaenoic acid, also known as EPA (an omega-3 fat). These two substances are the building blocks for the fatty acids that play a part in either promoting or reducing inflammation. Sears calls this comparison his "silent inflammation profile." Visit Nutrasource Diagnostics online at nutrasource.ca for information on where you can get your levels of these inflammation markers tested.

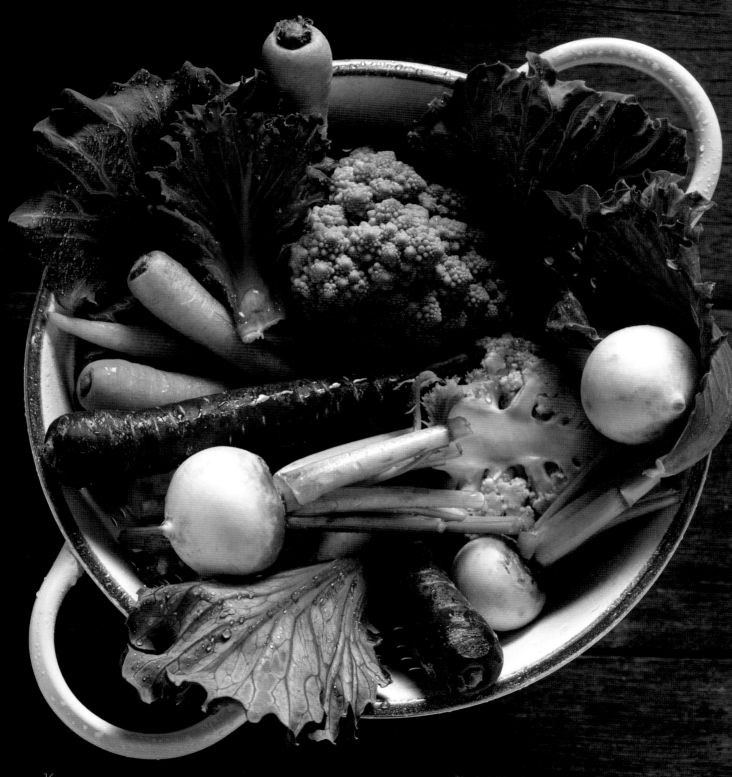

how to fight chronic inflammation

When most people feel the pain, swelling, and other common symptoms of chronic inflammation, their first impulse is to take medication, such as painkillers, antihistamines, or steroids, to combat their symptoms. Occasional use of anti-inflammatory drugs isn't associated with problems for the majority of people, but long-term use can cause side effects.

Nonsteroidal anti-inflammatory drugs (NSAIDs), such as ibuprofen and coxibs (Celebrex), work by interfering with COX-2 enzymes, which are needed to make prostaglandins, the inflammatory substances that cause pain and swelling. One of the most common side effects of these drugs is stomach bleeding. Less likely but still significant is the increased potential for heart attack, stroke, and liver and kidney problems. An alternative to using NSAIDs to treat inflammation with pain is to take acetaminophen, such as Tylenol. Acetaminophen carries less risk for side effects; however, it will only provide comfort and won't reduce the inflammation.

As the term suggests, antihistamines block the initial action of histamine, the first substance to participate in an inflammatory response. Antihistamines also block the activity of cytokines. Consequently, the drugs can be effective at the first signs of inflammation as well as hours later. H1-antihistamines interfere with the actions of histamine at H1-receptors and are commonly used to treat allergic rhinitis, allergic conjunctivitis, urticaria, coughs, and colds.

Corticosteroids, also known simply as "steroids," such as cortisone and prednisone, are sometimes prescribed to reduce inflammation. These drugs are synthetic substances similar to cortisol, and, like cortisol, they can tamp down an inflammatory response. They are administered by injection, taken orally, or applied topically. In cases of dangerous inflammation, steroids can be lifesaving. However, regular use of steroids, especially when taken orally, is usually accompanied by side effects, some of which can be serious. In addition to stomach bleeding, which NSAIDs also can cause, steroids weaken bone and tissue, promote bruising, increase weight gain, and exacerbate mood swings. People with osteoarthritis and uncontrolled diabetes or high blood pressure should be particularly careful to avoid steroids or take them only under close medical supervision.

NATURAL SOLUTIONS TO CURB INFLAMMATION

Instead of blocking the inflammatory process with potentially harmful medications, use diet and lifestyle to reduce the causes of inflammation and increase the factors that inhibit it naturally. Dietary improvements will have the greatest impact overall.

The Right Balance of Omega-3 Oils

Anti-inflammatory drugs as well as fish oil (which is high in omega-3 fatty acids) have been proven to reduce cancer risk. Fish oil has also been shown to slow the spread of prostate cancer. It's safe to assume that a diet high in omega-3 fats would be similarly protective. Omega-3 fatty acids might help encourage apoptosis (cell death) only in tumor cells but not in healthy cells and make cancer cells more receptive to chemotherapy.

There's some evidence that anti-inflammatory medications taken on a regular basis can lower the risk of Alzheimer's disease. That's also true of a diet high in omega-3 fats, so adhering to an anti-inflammatory diet could be equally protective. For instance, older people who eat the most fish develop Alzheimer's less frequently than those who don't. Interestingly, omega-3 fatty acids have an easier time crossing the brain barrier than many drugs do; the omega-3 fat DHA is a building block for brain tissue. DHA has shown promise in improving cognition in Alzheimer's patients and reducing the development of brain lesions in mice.

The standard Western diet tends to be very high in grains, particularly wheat, which tilts the balance of fatty acids toward omega-6s. It also contains limited amounts of vegetables, legumes, seeds, and nuts, which are rich in omega-3s. Farmed food animals and fish are also fed an overabundance of grains, rather than the grasses or algae they used to eat.

To achieve a healthy balance, Western populations would need to move away from the processed foods so prevalent in today's modern diets and consume two to four times as much omega-3 fatty acids as omega-6s. Research confirms that this ratio would still allow omega-3 fatty acids to access an adequate amount of the COX enzymes needed to make anti-inflammatory fats.

Many popular cooking oils, such as corn, safflower, and sunflower, are high in omega-6s. Better choices for cooking are extra-virgin olive oil and organic canola oil. Both still contain omega-6s but at much lower levels than most other oils. Although peanut oil and coconut oil are also very low in omega-6s, they contain no omega-3s. Oils that are high in omega-3s are flax, hemp, and walnut oils. Because omega-3 fats break down more easily in the presence of heat and light than omega-6s, store them in a cool, dark place or in the refrigerator, and do not heat or cook with them. Oils high in omega-3s are best used in salad dressings and cold spreads or drizzled over raw or warm cooked foods.

Nuts and seeds and their butters are also good sources of both types of essential fatty acids. Those that are high in omega-6s include pecans, pine nuts, pumpkin seeds, sesame seeds, and sunflower seeds. Nuts and seeds high in omega-3s or that have a better ratio of omega-3s to omega-6s include almonds, cashews, chia seeds, flaxseeds, hazelnuts, hemp seeds, peanuts (which actually are legumes, not tree nuts), pistachios, and walnuts. Those with the most omega-3s compared to omega-6s are chia seeds and flaxseeds. Walnuts contain more omega-3s per ounce than many other nuts, although they contain more omega-6s than chia seeds or flaxseeds.

It's difficult to chew whole flaxseeds adequately enough to break them down, so if they aren't ground before they're consumed, the whole seeds tend to pass through the body undigested. Because any whole food that's broken down will expose the omega-3s they contain to damaging heat and light, it's best to grind flaxseeds right before using them. Alternatively, store freshly ground flaxseeds in an airtight container in the refrigerator for up to three days or in the freezer for up to two months; the ground seeds can be used straight from the freezer without thawing.

The Power of Phytochemicals

Phytochemicals are biologically active, non-nutritive substances in plants that help protect the plants from predatory insects and disease. Not only do phytochemicals protect plants, but they also impart similar protective benefits to people who eat plants on a regular basis. It's been theorized that organic produce may be higher in phytochemicals than conventionally grown food because organically grown plants need to develop greater natural resistance since they aren't treated with insecticides and fungicides.

When whole foods are refined, they're often stripped of the parts of the plant that contain the most phytochemicals. Cooking can have a detrimental effect on some phytochemicals, but heat can also make other phytochemicals more bioavailable.

Rich colors in fruits and vegetables indicate the presence of phytochemicals. The phytochemicals that have been shown to have the most potential for fighting inflammation are carotenoids (found in green, orange, and red vegetables and fruits), flavonoids (found in berries, citrus fruits, and soy products), polyphenols (found in berries, grapes, green tea, and whole grains), and terpenes (found in cherries, the peels of citrus fruits, and rosemary). Certain spices that are rich in phytochemicals, such as black pepper and turmeric, have been shown to help curb inflammation. The phytochemicals in red wine and red grape juice (resveratrol), blue fruits (anthocyanins), and turmeric (curcumin) can reduce levels of prostaglandins and cytokines.

Although most phytochemicals are highly beneficial, a few, particularly alkaloids, might actually instigate inflammation in certain individuals. Alkaloids are present in vegetables in the nightshade family (eggplants, peppers, potatoes, and tomatoes), and some health advocates believe these foods exacerbate the painful symptoms of arthritis.

Avoid Trans Fats, Alcohol, and Caffeine

Don't consume foods that contain trans fats. These chemically altered fats inhibit the ability of COX enzymes to create anti-inflammatory prostaglandins. They also increase CRP (see page 4), especially in people who are overweight or obese.

Limit the use of alcohol and caffeine, both of which can reduce how much omega-3s can be used to create anti-inflammatory fats. However, because of the resveratrol in red wine, moderate amounts (up to two glasses per day for men or one glass per day for women) may offset any inflammatory activity promoted by alcohol.

Maintain a Healthy Weight

Inflammation has been shown to be higher in people who are overweight or obese. Body fat contains white blood cells, so an increase in weight increases the number of white blood cells releasing pro-inflammatory substances, which is directly correlated with a greater risk of diabetes. A diet based predominantly on a variety of whole plant foods, particularly fruits and vegetables, aids satiety, provides valuable fiber, and ensures a broad spectrum of inflammation fighters.

Limit Processed Foods

Avoid processed foods made with refined flours and instead eat intact whole grains. Replace sugar, sugary refined foods, and fruit juices with whole fresh fruits. A diet centered on foods that are naturally high in fiber reduces spikes in insulin levels more effectively than fiber supplements.

Consider adding naturally fermented foods to your diet. A growing body of evidence indicates that a healthy digestive system has a broad influence on overall wellness, beyond the organs of digestion. The intestines are home to a great many beneficial microorganisms, called probiotics, that convert nutrients and combat harmful microbial invaders. Naturally fermented sauerkraut and pickles are delicious sources of probiotics that help maintain a health-promoting digestive environment.

Include High-Protein Plant Foods

Many high-protein animal-derived foods—meat, poultry, and dairy products in particular—are sources of pro-inflammatory arachidonic acid. Although fatty fish can be a good source of omega-3 fatty acids, there are environmental concerns about our increasing reliance on fish as a protein source (see page 22).

Most people are surprised to learn that nearly all vegetables and even fruits contain small amounts of protein, so eating a wide variety of them will add to overall protein intake. High-protein whole plant foods, such as legumes (beans, lentils, and peas), nuts and seeds (particularly walnuts and flaxseeds, both of which are also high in omega-3s), and high-protein grains (such as amaranth, barley, Kamut, and oats) can easily replace animal protein in the diet. In addition to the common beans most people are familiar

FISH OIL: NOT THE BEST TOOL TO FIGHT INFLAMMATION

There's no question that fish oil, especially from oily cold-water fish, is an excellent source of the omega-3 fats that humans convert most easily into anti-inflammatory eicosanoids. However, the consumption of fish and their oil is problematic in several ways.

Common toxins in fish, including dioxin, mercury, PCBs, pesticides, and discarded pharmaceutical drugs, have become present in increasingly dangerous amounts in our oceans. Ingesting mercury at the levels often found in fish can cause neurological damage, while dioxin and PCBs have a host of adverse effects ranging from reduced fertility and immunity to heart problems. People who eat farmed fish instead of wild-caught fish in an attempt to avoid these contaminants might be surprised to learn that farmed fish often contain higher levels of dangerous chemicals than fish raised in ocean waters. That's because farmed fish are fed fish meal and oil from sea animals. Chemicals and toxins are stored in the fats of these animals and passed on to farmed fish in even higher concentrations than would occur in natural environments.

Even if these dangerous contaminants could be removed during processing, fish oil may not produce the results that claims suggest. Some studies show that large amounts of fish oil can increase the risk of colon cancer and may not have the protective effects against heart disease that was once believed. Other studies strongly dispute the claims that fish oil helps prevent Alzheimer's disease, cancer, and inflammation, or improves the immune system.

When weighing whether to consume fish oil, keep in mind the following two points: (1) Getting the right amount of essential fatty acids in order to reduce inflammation is a matter of balance, and taking high amounts of omega-3s is not necessarily a healthy practice. (2) The bounty of our oceans is at increased risk for depletion. The World Wildlife Fund estimates that the number of large ocean fish has decreased by about 80 percent over the last hundred years. Encouraging more people worldwide to consume increased amounts of fish and fish oil would ultimately make this situation more dire. Because fish farms rely on supplies of ocean fish as a source of feed, eating only farmed fish wouldn't relieve this serious problem.

The best alternative is to eat a diet that contains enough plant-based foods rich in omega-3 fatty acids to balance foods containing omega-6s. Freshly ground flaxseeds and chia seeds can be incorporated into cold cereals, salads, and smoothies. (Note that these seeds should be consumed shortly after grinding or stored for brief periods in the refrigerator or freezer to prevent degradation of their fragile oils.) Walnuts and dark leafy greens are also good sources of omega-3s. If you think you need additional omega-3 supplementation, consider getting it from the same source that ocean fish do: marine microalgae. Supplements made from microalgae are free of the toxins found in fish and untreated fish oils and supply omega-3 fats of the same quality.

with (such as chickpeas, kidney beans, and pinto beans), whole soy foods, including edamame and tempeh, are protein powerhouses.

There are many all-vegetable meat replacements in the marketplace, but these are best reserved for occasional treats rather relied upon as dietary staples. The additional ingredients and amount of processing necessary to manufacture these products often makes them less than ideal.

DESIGNING AN ANTI-INFLAMMATORY DIET

A variety of anti-inflammatory diets have been devised by popular physicians and nutrition writers. Nutritionist Monica Reinagel developed a rating system that ranks the inflammatory potential of hundreds of foods. Her system takes into account the amount and balance of nutrients in a food along with a number of other factors, including the following:

- the food's glycemic index (the potential of a food to raise blood glucose)
- the types of fat the food contains
- the amount of various antioxidants (such as vitamins C, E, and K, and certain B vitamins, as well as selenium and zinc) in the food
- how much of the amino acid homocysteine (a possible indicator of heart disease and Alzheimer's) the food contains

Use Reinagel's website (nutritiondata.self.com) to compare her rankings of various foods and determine which ones to emphasize in your diet and which ones to avoid.

The one drawback of using a ranking system is that it might encourage people to offset inflammation-inducing foods (such as meat and dairy products) with foods that have a low inflammation rating (such as cherries, chiles, and dark leafy greens). The best results will come from avoiding problem foods altogether and relying only on healthy ingredients.

Andrew Weil, MD, has drawn up recommendations for an anti-inflammatory diet in his book *Healthy Aging*. Rather than zeroing in on particular foods, Weil encourages sufficient water intake and provides suggestions for calorie and fiber consumption as well as amounts and types of carbohydrates, fats, protein, and supplements (including particular phytochemicals, vitamins, and minerals).

Each plan has minor variances and presents somewhat conflicting recommendations. Evaluate them individually to determine which one will work best for you.

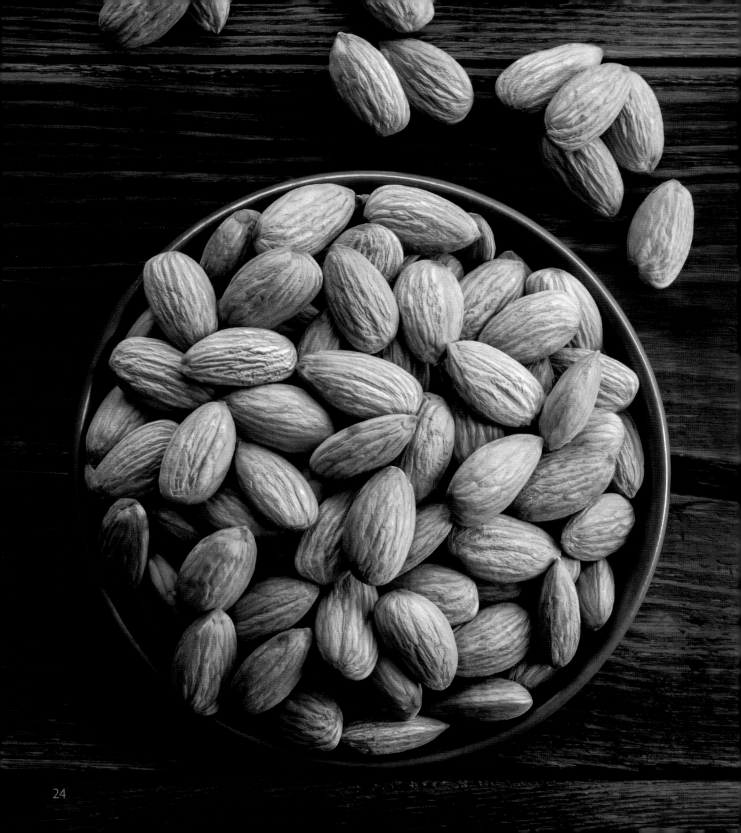

anti-inflammatory foods, nutrients, and supplements

You'll find many delicious, easy-to-prepare recipes in this book to help you maximize the benefits of inflammation-fighting foods. Nuts and seeds rich in omega-3 fatty acids provide the most protection, but a wide variety of vegetables and fruits also contribute supportive nutrients. The information that follows will highlight these foods and explain how they keep inflammation at bay.

ANTI-INFLAMMATORY SEEDS, NUTS, AND OILS

Many seeds and nuts are anti-inflammatory, either because they're particularly high in omega-3s or they contain substantial amounts of other nutrients shown to decrease inflammation.

Chia seeds and **flaxseeds** have some of the highest amounts of omega-3 fatty acids in the plant kingdom, with over 7 grams in one tablespoon of flaxseed oil and 5 grams in two tablespoons of chia seeds. **Hemp seed oil** contains almost 3 grams per tablespoon. **Walnuts** not only contain more than 2 grams per ounce but also contain phytonutrients, such as juglone and tellimagrandin (a tannin), that might fight cancers of the breast and prostate as well as inflammation in general.

Almonds were shown in a Spanish study to decrease C-reactive protein (CRP) and other markers of inflammation. **Cashews** are high in copper and magnesium, which can help control free radicals and prevent bone loss, especially in people with rheumatoid arthritis. **Coconut** (which could be thought of as either a fruit or a nut) contains medium-chain fatty acids that fight viruses and reduce inflammation. A Brazilian study found that the monounsaturated fatty acids in **macadamia oil** helped block inflammatory activity promoted by fatty tissue.

Be aware that certain nuts might cause inflammation, particularly in people who have an allergy or intolerance to tree nuts or peanuts. An intolerance may cause mild chronic inflammation but not be troublesome enough to arouse suspicion that nuts are the culprit. If you have digestive difficulties, try eliminating nuts from your diet to determine whether they could be the source of the problem.

ANTI-INFLAMMATORY FRUITS

Berries

Blueberries, cherries, cranberries, raspberries, and strawberries contain phytochemicals called anthocyanins that have been shown to reduce several substances involved in the inflammatory response. Anthocyanins give these fruits their rich blue, purple, and red colors.

Research from Harvard University demonstrated that anthocyanins can lower heart attack risk by about one-third, particularly in women under fifty. According to research done at Oregon Health & Science University in 2012, tart cherries may have the highest anti-inflammatory potential of any food because of their anthocyanin content, and these levels may provide pain protection that's equal to some NSAIDs. Another study published in the *Journal of Nutrition* found that eating about one-half pound of sweet cherries per day reduced CRP levels.

Cranberries and strawberries contain significant amounts of polyphenols, another group of antioxidant phytochemicals that fight inflammation by reducing the buildup of platelets in blood vessels and lowering blood pressure. Strawberries also contain a natural anti-inflammatory called quercetin that protects against heart disease. In addition, the high amount of vitamin C in strawberries helps protect against asthma.

Açaí berries are small red berries native to South America and Brazil, and dried açaí berries have become popular worldwide for their nutritional content. A study conducted by Sloan Kettering Memorial Cancer Center found that açaí berries might suppress interleukins and COX enzymes.

Goji berries are bright red berries from Asia that have traditionally been used to promote longevity and vitality. Their active anti-inflammatory ingredient, beta-sitosterol, reduces the risk of heart disease, lowers cholesterol, and has a positive effect on enlarged prostates in men. See the box on page 28 for more information about goji berries.

Citrus Fruits

In addition to the vitamin C that's found in **lemons, limes, and oranges**, citrus fruits also contain limonoids. These phytochemicals slow the growth of breast cancer cells as well as colon, lung, and skin cancer cells.

Tropical Fruits

The leaves of the **guava** tree were the subject of a recent Korean study and were shown to reduce prostaglandins and COX-2 enzymes. Guava fruit is high in the antioxidants vitamin C and lycopene.

Succulent, green **kiwifruit** is high in vitamin C. It also contains a peptide called kissper that has demonstrated potential to reduce infections associated with colon disease, specifically Crohn's disease. Note that individuals with allergies to latex should eat kiwifruit with caution, as antibodies to latex can react to the protein in kiwifruit (as well as to the protein in avocados and bananas) the same as they do to latex.

Tropical **papaya** is rich in vitamins C and E. Papaya fruit has been shown to heal surface wounds, reduce oxidative damage, and increase the activity of antioxidant enzymes. Fresh **pineapple** contains bromelain, a mixture of protein-digesting enzymes that decreases cytokines and slows down the action of leukocytes to an injury site. It may prohibit the formation of cancer by dissolving the protective protein layer that surrounds tumor cells. Research done at Duke University found that both fresh and frozen pineapple were effective at decreasing the incidence and severity of inflammatory bowel disease. Bromelain has also been used to reduce inflammation from arthritis, sinusitis, sprains and strains, and surgery.

Other Fruits

A study done at Florida State University showed that eating an **apple** daily can decrease amounts of CRP by up to 30 percent. The fats in **avocados** help improve the absorption and effectiveness of carotenoids, substances

NIGHTSHADE FRUITS AND VEGETABLES: ARTHRITIS FRIENDS OR FOES?

Nightshades are a group of plants that comprise a number of popular vegetables and fruits, such as **eggplants**, **goji berries**, **okra**, **peppers** (including **bell**, **cayenne**, **chile**, and **paprika**), **potatoes**, **tomatillos**, and **tomatoes**. Many of these foods contain high amounts of antioxidants, such as vitamin C and carotenoids (especially beta-carotene and lycopene). Chiles (hot peppers) are a source of capsaicin, a compound that is often used topically for pain relief.

Despite these benefits, many people believe that nightshade vegetables and fruits provoke inflammation (especially arthritis) instead of subduing it. Educated opinions about this are equally divided. The US Food and Drug Administration has stated that solanine, an alkaloid found in a number of nightshade foods, is poorly absorbed and therefore unlikely to be implicated as a cause of arthritis. However, a number of patients with arthritis have reported anecdotal evidence of a link between eating nightshades and an increase in the severity of their symptoms.

Since nightshade foods affect people differently, arthritis sufferers might want to eliminate them from their diets for a trial period of up to three months. After the elimination period, the foods can be reintroduced gradually, one at a time, to determine if any of them trigger or exacerbate symptoms.

that can inhibit the formation of inflammatory cytokines. **Rhubarb** has been shown to fight cytokines involved with systemic inflammation and may also be effective at healing cold sores and improving kidney function. (Note that eating too much rhubarb can cause diarrhea and stomach cramps. Also, rhubarb is not recommended in large amounts for anyone with a history of kidney stones.)

ANTI-INFLAMMATORY VEGETABLES

Allium Vegetables

The allium family contains a number of pungent vegetables, such as **garlic**, **leeks**, **onions**, and **shallots**, that are known for reducing inflammation. Biochemists in South Africa determined that the sulfur-containing compounds in garlic may help stimulate the immune system to fight cancer, while Iranian researchers found that fresh onion juice reduced both acute and chronic pain related to inflammation.

Cruciferous Vegetables

Bok choy, **Brussels sprouts**, **cabbage**, **cauliflower**, **chard**, **collard greens**, **kale**, **mustard greens**, and **turnips** are part of the cruciferous family of vegetables. As a group, they're potent inflammation fighters. In general, they're high in vitamin C as well as other phytonutrients and antioxidants. A 2006 study from the Feinstein Institute for Medical Research showed that choline, a compound found in cauliflower, suppressed inflammation. A number of researchers, especially in Poland, have been studying the potential of sauerkraut (fermented cabbage) to fight the growth of cancer. **Turnip greens** are a good source of vitamin K, an inflammation regulator, and omega-3 fatty acids, the building blocks for inflammation fighters most often found in nuts and seeds.

Root Vegetables

Betanin, one of the most researched betalains, a class of antioxidant pigments, gives **beets** a high concentration of detoxifying substances that fight inflammation. **Beet greens** are also high in vitamins A, C, and K. The bright orange color of **carrots** comes from beta-carotene, which the body converts to vitamin A. Beta-carotene lowers inflammatory markers, particularly interleukin-6. **Rutabaga** is a good source of inulin, a substance that promotes the growth of beneficial digestive bacteria and a healthy immune system.

Jicama is a root vegetable popular in Mexican cuisine that is often prepared like potatoes. However, jicama contains fewer starches per serving than potatoes. As a result, it causes less of a spike in blood glucose levels and is less of a driver of inflammation. **Sweet potatoes** contain beta-carotene, fiber, manganese, and vitamins B_6 and C. Purple sweet potato extract has been shown to reduce inflammation. Sweet potatoes are an excellent alternative to white potatoes in most recipes.

Squash

The squash family encompasses a number of inflammation-fighting vegetables, including **summer squashes** (such as **zucchini**), **pumpkins**, **winter squashes**, and even **cucumbers**. In general, squashes are high in vitamin C, and orange squashes and pumpkins are high in beta-carotene. Cucumbers contain lignans that can reduce cancer risk and have been shown to block proteins that increase inflammation.

Other Vegetables

Celery is particularly rich in antioxidants, as it contains flavanols as well as the polyphenols caffeic acid and ferulic acid. **Celeriac (celery root)** is a source of vitamin C. Celery also is a good source of silicon, and both celery and celeriac contain vitamin K; these nutrients help maintain the health of joints and connective tissues.

Eating **mushrooms** is a gentle, noninvasive way to prevent metastatic cancer tumors and enhance the action of chemotherapy. White button mushrooms in particular have been shown to increase the formation of macrophages, the white blood cells that attack harmful invading microbes.

The protective power of olive trees can be found in **olive leaves**, **olives**, and **olive oil**, which is pressed from olives. Two phenolic compounds in olives, hydroxytyrosol and oleuropein, have been shown to help fight cardiovascular disease.

Consuming **soy foods** helps to reduce amounts of interleukin as well as tumor necrosis factor, a cytokine found during systemic inflammation. Whole soy foods, such as **edamame**, **tempeh**, and **tofu**, are more protective than highly processed soy foods. **Spinach** is a good source of the inflammation fighters carotenes and flavonoids. Spinach is also rich in the B vitamin folate and a number of minerals, including calcium, iron, magnesium, and potassium.

OTHER FOODS AND BEVERAGES

Chocolate

Raw cacao powder is packed with antioxidants that slow inflammation, and these nutritious substances are more readily available in chocolate made with little or no added fat. Scientists now believe that beneficial bacteria in the large intestine convert the antioxidants in chocolate for use in fighting inflammation, but they caution that highly processed chocolate (even very dark chocolate) is not as effective as raw, unprocessed cacao.

Green Tea

The teas most people are familiar with (black and green) come from the same *Camellia sinensis* plant; the differences are due to how each type of tea is processed. Green tea contains more flavonoids, particularly catechins, than black tea, and therefore has a greater effect on inflammation.

ANTI-INFLAMMATORY HERBS AND SPICES

The concentrated oil from **basil** was shown in an Indian study to significantly reduce joint swelling in just one day. Researchers found that eugenol, the substance that gives basil its distinctive aroma, had similar benefits as several anti-inflammatory drugs but without the gastrointestinal side effects. **Oregano** contains carvacrol, an antioxidant that fights both inflammation and microbial infections, and rosmarinic acid, which helps protect against cancer. **Parsley** is a good source of myricetin, a phenol that blocks COX-2 enzymes and cytokines, and apigenin, a flavone that helps to fight cancerous cells without harming surrounding tissue. **Peppermint** has antimicrobial properties.

The coriander plant can be used as an herb (**cilantro**) or a spice (**coriander seeds**). Both the fresh plant and seeds protect against inflammatory diseases that attack the nervous system, such as Alzheimer's and Parkinson's.

The spice that gives Indian food its distinctive yellow color is **turmeric**. It has a historic use in folk medicine as a pain reliever, and recent studies support the action of its active ingredient, curcumin, against COX-2 inhibitors. Piperine is the active ingredient in **black pepper** that provides its characteristic pungency. Researchers at Hamdard University in New Delhi found piperine to be extremely helpful in reducing the symptoms of rheumatoid arthritis. Piperine also helps the body assimilate certain medications and supplements and is recommended as a companion supplement to the curcumin in turmeric.

In studies of mice, extracts of **cardamom** reduced precancerous cells. The eucalyptol in cardamom was also shown to reduce gastrointestinal inflammation in rats. **Cinnamon** gets its flavor and aroma from a flavonoid called cinnamaldehyde. This substance will fight the growth of leukemia and melanoma cells and overall tumor growth. The anti-inflammatory effects of the active

THE CURATIVE POWER OF CURRY POWDER

Curry powder, the distinctive ingredient in many Indian foods, can be a potent anti-inflammatory. The powder, which generally varies from household to household and cook to cook, is a mixture of many different inflammation-fighting spices, such as black pepper, coriander, cumin, ginger, mustard, and turmeric.

ingredients in **ginger**—namely gingerol and zingerone—have been widely studied. They've been shown to reduce prostaglandins, COX enzymes, and leukotrienes, particularly in relation to infection and cancer.

USING ANTI-INFLAMMATORY FOODS

The best way to increase your consumption of anti-inflammatory foods is by using recipes that incorporate these foods as ingredients. In fact, it's easy to make dishes that include half a dozen or more different inflammation fighters at once. At the same time, it's a good idea to choose recipes that limit the use of foods that promote inflammation.

Plant-based dishes are strong in both regards. When fruits and vegetables are emphasized, dishes will automatically include many types of produce that contain inflammation-fighting compounds. In addition, using plant protein instead of meat, eggs, and dairy products essentially eliminates the inflammation-causing substances found in animal foods.

The recipes that follow are some of my favorites, and they're all inherently health promoting. To help you identify **the ingredients that fight inflammation,** I've highlighted those items in the ingredient lists. The smoothies not only showcase nutritious fruits, but also nuts and nut milks, seeds, power-packed supplements, and even vegetables. Find alternatives to bacon and eggs in the breakfast recipes, and feast on an array of fresh veggies in the salad section. I'll show you how to make a few naturally fermented foods as well as some delicious alternatives to dairy-based sauces and toppings. You'll never miss meat with these warming soups and hearty main dishes; even my desserts employ ingredients rich in anti-inflammatory ingredients. Enjoy these recipes just as they're presented or use them as an inspiration for adding inflammation-fighting foods to your own favorite dishes.

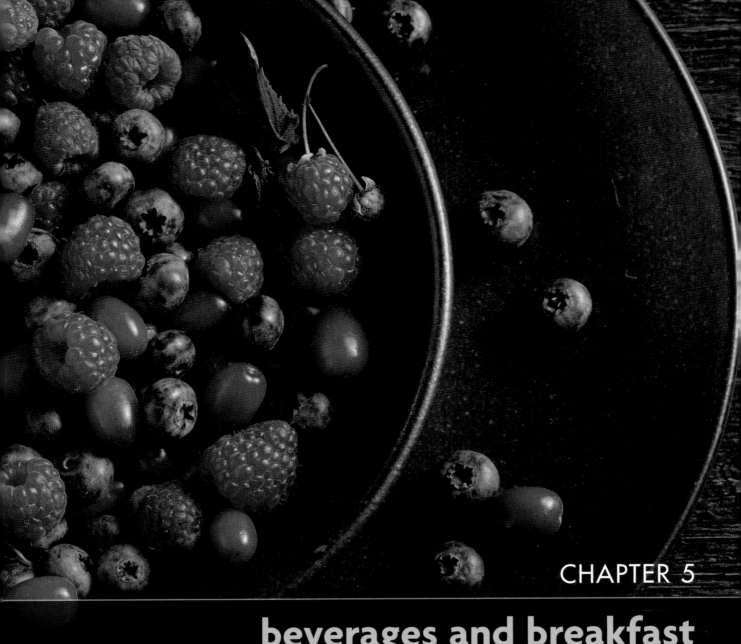

beverages and breakfast

golden milk TEA

MAKES 4 SERVINGS

Per serving:

50 calories

0 g protein

5 g fat (0 g sat)

14 g carbs

5 mg sodium

220 mg calcium

1 g fiber

Curcumin is the primary beneficial compound found in the spice turmeric. To increase the body's absorption of curcumin, turmeric is often combined with black pepper. Because curcumin is fat soluble, cooking it in oil or combining it with high-fat foods, such as the coconut milk used in this creamy beverage, will increase its bioavailability.

> 4 cups plain or vanilla **coconut milk** beverage or **almond milk**
> 1½ teaspoons ground **turmeric**
> 1 teaspoon ground **ginger**
> ¾ teaspoon ground **cinnamon**
> Pinch freshly ground **black pepper**
> Agave nectar or maple syrup

Put the milk, turmeric, ginger, cinnamon, and pepper in a medium sauce-pan and stir to combine. Cook over medium heat, stirring occasionally, until hot but not boiling, about 5 minutes. Sweeten with agave nectar as desired. Serve immediately. Store leftover tea in an airtight container in the refrigerator.

Note: Analysis doesn't include freshly ground black pepper or agave nectar.

berry blast-off SMOOTHIE

Start your morning with a blast of energy from this smoothie. It's bursting with blue, purple, or red berries, along with other colorful fruits and veggies, which are all blended with omega-rich hemp and chia seeds.

MAKES 2 SERVINGS

Per serving:

221 calories

8 g protein

6 g fat (1 g sat)

40 g carbs

51 mg sodium

85 mg calcium

7 g fiber

1 cup water

1 cup fresh or frozen mixed **berries** (such as blueberries, raspberries, or strawberries)

2 large leaves red curly or Russian **kale**, stemmed

1 large maroon **carrot**, sliced, or 1 small red **beet**, peeled and diced

½ cup **grape juice** or **pomegranate juice**

½ cup fresh or frozen pitted sweet or sour **cherries**

¼ cup **goji berries** or dried **cranberries**

2 tablespoons **hemp seeds**

2 teaspoons **chia seeds**

Put all the ingredients in a blender and process until smooth. Scrape down the blender jar and process for 15 seconds longer. Serve immediately.

TIP: If you're using only fresh fruit and would like a frozen smoothie, add ½ cup of ice cubes.

nutty chocolate SMOOTHIE

MAKES 2 SERVINGS

Per serving:

404 calories

13 g protein

20 g fat (3 g sat)

51 g carbs

159 mg sodium

296 mg calcium

8 g fiber

The combination of chocolate and nuts is beloved by young and old alike. The flavor of bananas pairs perfectly with both these ingredients and adds a sweet, creamy base to this ultrarich, liquid confection.

1½ cups **chocolate nondairy milk**

2 **bananas,** broken into chunks

½ **cup ice cubes**

3 tablespoons **almond butter** or other **nut butter**

1½ tablespoons **cacao powder** or unsweetened cocoa powder

1 tablespoon ground **flaxseeds** or **flaxseed meal**

½ **teaspoon vanilla extract**

Pinch **sea salt**

Put all the ingredients in a blender and process until smooth. Scrape down the blender jar and process for 15 seconds longer. Serve immediately.

go green tea SMOOTHIE

Adding leafy greens to a smoothie is a painless way to get more greens into your diet. Affectionately called green smoothies by aficionados, they're also an excellent means to incorporate other healthy ingredients. This one is made with a combination of green-colored fruits and veggies and green tea to energize your morning or keep you going after a workout.

2 cups stemmed baby **spinach**, **kale**, or other **leafy greens**, lightly packed

1 cup seedless white **grapes**

1 cup cold **green tea**

1 Granny Smith **apple**, cored and diced

1 Hass **avocado**, diced

⅔ cup diced **cucumber**

1 large stalk **celery**, sliced

½ cup ice cubes

¼ cup fresh **mint** leaves, lightly packed

2 tablespoons **hemp seeds**, or 2 teaspoons **chia seeds**

Juice of ½ **lemon**

Put all the ingredients in a blender and process until smooth. Scrape down the blender jar and process for 15 seconds longer. Serve immediately.

MAKES 2 SERVINGS

Per serving:

285 calories

6 g protein

16 g fat (2 g sat)

35 g carbs

51 mg sodium

67 mg calcium

10 g fiber

superfood smoothie BOWL

MAKES 1 SERVING

Per serving:

607 calories

15 g protein

24 g fat (3 g sat)

92 g carbs

200 mg sodium

396 mg calcium

19 g fiber

Swap your straw for a spoon! Take your smoothie to the next level by transforming it into an eye-catching smoothie bowl. Simply make your smoothie extra thick, pour it into a large bowl, and garnish it with your favorite crunchy and chewy toppings along with additional fresh or frozen berries or diced fruit.

1 frozen **banana**, broken into chunks

1 cup stemmed **leafy greens**, lightly packed

½ cup plain nondairy milk

1 tablespoon **nut** or **seed butter**

1 teaspoon **chia seeds**

1 teaspoon ground **flaxseeds** or **flaxseed meal**

1 package (2 ounces) frozen **açaí purée**, or 1 teaspoon **açaí powder**

1 teaspoon spirulina or chlorella powder (optional)

½ cup diced or sliced **fruit**, ⅓ cup fresh **berries**, or 2 tablespoons **pomegranate seeds**

2 tablespoons whole or diced dried **fruit**

2 tablespoons coarsely chopped nuts, or 1 tablespoon raw seeds

Put the banana, leafy greens, milk, nut butter, chia seeds, flaxseeds, açaí purée, and optional spirulina powder in a blender and process until smooth. Scrape down the blender jar and process for 15 seconds longer. The mixture should be very thick, with a consistency similar to soft-serve ice cream.

Transfer to a bowl and top with the fresh fruit, dried fruit, and nuts. Serve immediately.

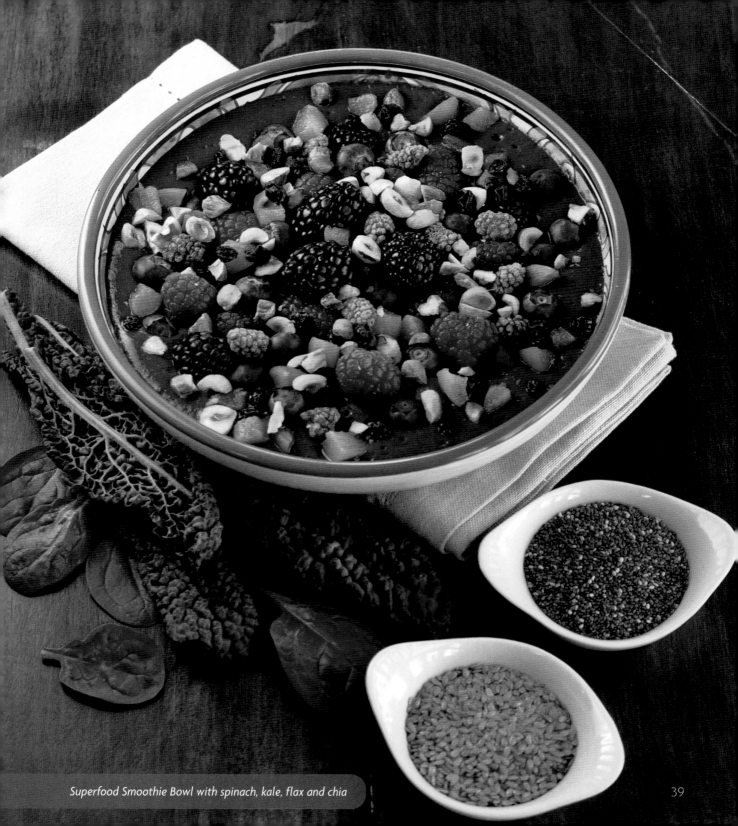

Superfood Smoothie Bowl with spinach, kale, flax and chia

39

STEEL-CUT oats porridge

MAKES 4 SERVINGS

Per serving:

365 calories

11 g protein

15 g fat (1 g sat)

51 g carbs

217 mg sodium

201 mg calcium

7 g fiber

To create steel-cut oats, a steel burr mill is used to cut whole oat groats into small pieces. For a praiseworthy pot of porridge, oatmeal enthusiasts often opt for steel-cut rather than rolled oats. To make a chilled, no-cook version, try the variation that follows.

1½ cups water

1½ cups plain **almond milk** or other nondairy milk

¼ teaspoon sea salt

1 cup steel-cut oats

¾ cup dried **fruit** (such as **cranberries**, currants, or raisins)

½ cup raw **sunflower** or **hemp seeds**

3 tablespoons ground **flaxseeds** or **flaxseed meal**

Ground **cinnamon** (optional)

Maple syrup (optional)

Put the water, milk, and salt in a medium saucepan and bring to a boil over high heat. Add the oats and dried fruit and stir to combine. Decrease the heat to low and cook, stirring occasionally, until the mixture thickens and the oats are cooked to your liking, 10 to 15 minutes. Remove from the heat.

Add the sunflower seeds and flaxseeds and stir until evenly distributed. Garnish each serving with cinnamon and maple syrup if desired.

> **NO-COOK OVERNIGHT OATS:** Put 1¾ cups nondairy milk, 1 cup plain or vanilla nondairy yogurt (preferably Greek-style), 1 cup steel-cut oats, 3 table-spoons nut or seed butter, and 1 teaspoon vanilla extract in a large bowl and stir to combine. Cover and refrigerate for 8 to 12 hours. Stir well before serving. Top with chopped fresh or thawed frozen fruit or berries and chopped nuts or seeds as desired. Makes 4 servings.

blender oat PANCAKES

Briefly toasting steel-cut oats intensifies their flavor. For this recipe, a trusty blender transforms the cooled oats into a wholesome flour, which in turn is blended with other pantry staples to create a thick pancake batter. Serve the pancakes with your favorite toppings, such as jam, vegan butter, maple or fruit-based syrup, or sliced fresh fruit or berries.

2 cups steel-cut oats

1⅔ cups plain or vanilla nondairy milk

1½ tablespoons lemon juice or cider vinegar

1 tablespoon ground flaxseeds or flaxseed meal

1 teaspoon baking powder

1 teaspoon vanilla extract

¾ teaspoon ground cinnamon

½ teaspoon baking soda

½ teaspoon sea salt

MAKES 8 PANCAKES

Per pancake:

149 calories

6 g protein

4 g fat (0.5 g sat)

23 g carbs

264 mg sodium

113 mg calcium

3 g fiber

Put the oats in a large, dry skillet and cook over medium heat, stirring occasionally, until lightly toasted and fragrant, about 3 minutes. Remove from the heat. Let cool completely, about 10 minutes.

Transfer the cooled oats to a blender and process into a fine flour, about 1 minute. Add the milk, lemon juice, flaxseeds, baking powder, vanilla extract, cinnamon, baking soda, and salt and process until smooth. Scrape down the blender jar and process for 15 seconds longer. Let the batter rest for 5 minutes.

Lightly oil a large cast-iron or nonstick skillet or griddle or mist with cooking spray. Heat over medium heat. When the skillet is hot, portion the batter into it, using ⅓ cup of batter for each pancake. Cook until the edges of the pancakes are dry and the bottoms are lightly browned, 3 to 4 minutes. Flip the pancakes over and cook until lightly browned on the other side, 2 to 3 minutes.

Lightly oil the skillet between batches and repeat with the remaining batter. Serve hot.

PALEO grits

MAKES 4 SERVINGS

Per serving:

369 calories

14 g protein

32 g fat (3 g sat)

13 g carbs

459 mg sodium

120 mg calcium

7 g fiber

For generations in the US South, hot grits have been served as part of a hearty break-fast. This recipe throws tradition to the wind by using almond flour or almond meal instead of the traditional corn grits, but it's just as thick, creamy, and delicious.

3 cups water

¾ teaspoon sea salt

2 cups **almond flour** or **almond meal**

2 tablespoons nutritional yeast flakes

1½ tablespoons vegan butter

Hot sauce (optional)

Put the water and salt in a medium saucepan and bring to a boil over high heat. Slowly whisk in the almond flour. Decrease the heat to low and simmer, whisking occasionally, until the mixture is thick and creamy, 10 to 15 minutes. Stir in the nutritional yeast and butter until evenly distributed. Garnish with hot sauce if desired. Serve hot.

> **PALEO GRITS WITH GREEN ONIONS AND CHILES:** After whisking the almond flour into the water, add ½ cup thinly sliced green onions and 2 jalapeño chiles, cut in half lengthwise, seeded, and thinly sliced.

> **PALEO GRITS WITH GREENS:** Put 3 cups stemmed and coarsely chopped kale or spinach, lightly packed, 1 tablespoon minced garlic, and 1½ teaspoons olive oil in large cast-iron or nonstick skillet and cook over medium-high heat, stirring occasionally, for 5 minutes. Top the cooked grits with the greens.

indian-style tofu SCRAMBLE

In this vegan version of scrambled eggs, curry powder adds both flavor and a yellow tint to crumbled tofu, which is cooked along with red onion, tomatoes, and spinach.

1 pound extra-firm **tofu**

2 tablespoons nutritional yeast flakes

1 tablespoon reduced-sodium tamari

1 teaspoon **curry powder**, or ½ teaspoon ground **turmeric**

½ cup diced red **onion**

1 tablespoon minced **garlic**

1 tablespoon **coconut oil** or other oil

1 cup diced **tomatoes**

3 cups baby **spinach**, lightly packed

¼ cup chopped fresh **cilantro**, lightly packed

Sea salt

Freshly ground **black pepper**

MAKES 4 SERVINGS

Per serving:

236 calories

21 g protein

14 g fat (5 g sat)

8 g carbs

162 mg sodium

164 mg calcium

2 g fiber

Crumble the tofu into a small bowl using your fingers. Add the nutritional yeast, tamari, and curry powder and stir until well combined.

Put the onion, garlic, and oil in a large cast-iron or nonstick skillet and cook over medium-high heat, stirring occasionally, for 2 minutes. Add the tofu mixture and tomatoes and cook, stirring occasionally, for 8 minutes.

Add the spinach and cilantro and cook, stirring occasionally, until the spinach has wilted and the other vegetables are tender, 1 to 2 minutes. Season with salt and pepper to taste. Serve hot.

Note: Analysis doesn't include sea salt or freshly ground black pepper.

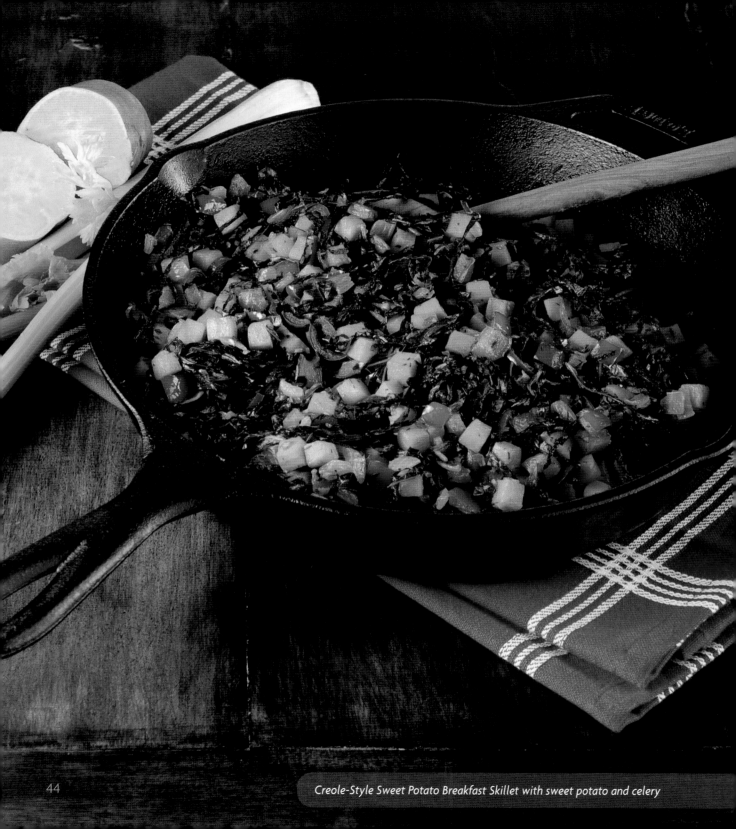

Creole-Style Sweet Potato Breakfast Skillet with sweet potato and celery

creole-style sweet potato BREAKFAST SKILLET

In the Creole cuisine of Louisiana, the combination of bell pepper, celery, and onion is commonly referred to as the "holy trinity." This flavor-enhancing blend unites with sweet potatoes, collard greens, and green onions in this breakfast skillet, along with some jalapeño chiles and cayenne for a little heat to round out the flavors.

MAKES 4 SERVINGS

Per serving:

205 calories

5 g protein

4 g fat (1 g sat)

32 g carbs

55 mg sodium

116 mg calcium

12 g fiber

1 cup diced red or yellow **bell pepper**

1 cup diced yellow **onion**

2 stalks **celery**, diced

2 tablespoons **olive oil**

2½ cups peeled and finely diced **sweet potatoes**

½ cup thinly sliced **green onions**

2 jalapeño **chiles**, cut in half lengthwise, seeded, and thinly sliced

1 tablespoon minced **garlic**

1½ teaspoons dried thyme

½ teaspoon **cayenne**

2 cups stemmed and thinly sliced **collard greens**, lightly packed

Sea salt

Freshly ground **black pepper**

Put the bell pepper, onion, celery, and oil in a large cast-iron or nonstick skillet and cook over medium-high heat, stirring occasionally, for 5 minutes. Add the sweet potatoes and cook, stirring occasionally, for 8 minutes.

Add the green onions, chiles, garlic, thyme, and cayenne and cook, stirring occasionally, for 2 minutes. Add the collard greens and cook, stirring occasionally, until the greens have wilted and the other vegetables are tender, 3 to 5 minutes. Season with salt and pepper to taste. Serve hot.

Note: Analysis doesn't include sea salt or freshly ground black pepper.

red flannel HASH

MAKES 4 SERVINGS

Per serving:

75 calories

5 g protein

3 g fat (0.4 g sat)

11 g carbs

259 mg sodium

151 mg calcium

6 g fiber

Savory breakfast hash is traditionally made from coarsely chopped leftover meat, potatoes, and other vegetables. When beets replace some of the potatoes, the dish is referred to as a red flannel hash, as in this plant-based version, which uses mushrooms instead of meat.

1 pound red **beets** with greens

2 cups (4 ounces) coarsely chopped button or crimini **mushrooms**

1 cup finely diced red or yellow **onion**

2 tablespoons **olive oil**

1½ tablespoons minced **garlic**

1½ teaspoons dried **basil**

1½ teaspoons **chili powder**

1½ teaspoons dried thyme

1 tablespoon nutritional yeast flakes

Sea salt

Freshly ground **black pepper**

Cut the greens from the beets and coarsely chop the stems and leaves. Peel the beets and cut them into ¼-inch dice.

Put the mushrooms, onion, and oil in a large cast-iron or nonstick skillet and cook over medium-high heat, stirring occasionally, for 7 minutes. Add the beets and cook, stirring occasionally, for 10 minutes.

Add the beet stems and leaves, garlic, basil, chili powder, and thyme and cook, stirring occasionally, until the vegetables are tender, 7 to 8 minutes. Add the nutritional yeast and stir until evenly distributed. Season with salt and pepper to taste. Serve hot.

Note: Analysis doesn't include sea salt or freshly ground black pepper.

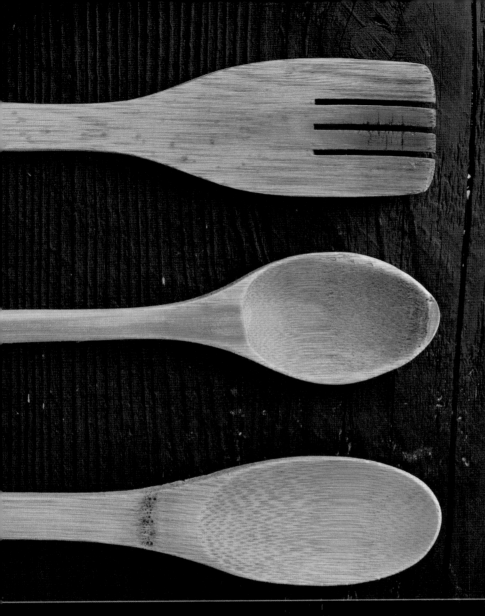

fermented foods, sauces, and spreads

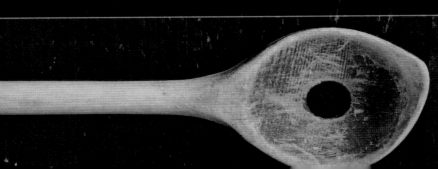

sauerkraut

MAKES 4 CUPS

Per ½ cup:

28 calories

2 g protein

0 g fat (0 g sat)

7 g carbs

873 mg sodium

45 mg calcium

3 g fiber

A few minutes of work plus a few days for fermenting will transform a humble head of cabbage into a batch of tangy sauerkraut. Enjoy it as a side dish or a topping for salads or sandwiches.

> 1 **head** (about 2 pounds) **cabbage**
> 1 tablespoon caraway seeds
> 1 tablespoon sea salt or pickling salt

Remove two outer leaves of the cabbage and set aside. Cut the remaining cabbage into quarters, cut out and discard the core, and thinly slice the cabbage crosswise. Transfer to a large bowl. Sprinkle the caraway seeds and salt over the cabbage and let rest for 5 minutes. Using your hands, vigorously massage the mixture until the cabbage begins to wilt and takes on a slightly cooked texture, 8 to 10 minutes.

Transfer the cabbage and any accumulated liquid to a 1-quart or larger jar or airtight container. Use the back of a spoon to firmly pack down the cabbage and remove any air bubbles. Completely cover the cabbage with the two reserved outer leaves and pack them down firmly using the back of a spoon.

Cover the jar with a clean towel and secure with a rubber band. Let rest at room temperature, away from direct sunlight, for 24 hours. Occasionally during the resting period firmly pack down the cabbage using the back of a spoon. Let the sauerkraut ferment for 3 to 10 days, or until the desired flavor is achieved. Remove and discard the layer of outer cabbage leaves. Cover the jar with a lid and store the sauerkraut in the refrigerator for up to 2 months.

> **VARIATIONS:** Replace the caraway seeds with 1½ teaspoons dried dill weed, 1 tablespoon grated horseradish, or 1½ tablespoons minced garlic or jalapeño chile.

This recipe proves that you don't need to master the canning process to make excellent homemade pickles. All you really need are patience and a fridge.

MAKES 15 SLICES

Per slice:

4 calories

0 g protein

0 g fat (0 g sat)

1 g carbs

38 mg sodium

40 mg calcium

0 g fiber

3 Kirby or other small **cucumbers** (about ½ pound)

¾ cup cider vinegar or white vinegar

½ cup water

1 tablespoon minced **garlic**

1 tablespoon chopped fresh dill, or 1 teaspoon dried dill weed

2 teaspoons unbleached cane sugar

2 teaspoons sea salt or pickling salt

1 teaspoon whole **black peppercorns**

1 teaspoon whole **coriander seeds** or **mustard seeds**

Cut off both ends of each cucumber and discard. Cut each cucumber lengthwise into ¼-inch-thick slices. Put the slices in a 1-pint or larger jar or airtight container and set aside.

Put the remaining ingredients in a small saucepan and stir to combine. Bring to a boil over high heat. Decrease the heat to low and simmer for 5 minutes. Pour the vinegar mixture into the jar and let cool completely. Cover the jar with a lid and store the pickles in the refrigerator for up to 2 months. The pickles will be ready to serve after 24 hours.

SPICY PICKLES: Replace the coriander seeds with ¼ teaspoon crushed red pepper flakes.

VARIATION: Cut the cucumbers lengthwise into spears or crosswise into ¼-inch-thick slices.

CASHEW cheese sauce

MAKES 3 CUPS

Per ¼ cup:

102 calories

6 g protein

6 g fat (1 g sat)

7 g carbs

143 mg sodium

7 mg calcium

2 g fiber

Both the color and flavor of this cheesy-tasting, cashew-based sauce are enhanced by the addition of paprika and an orange or yellow bell pepper. Pour this sauce over casseroles or stove-top dishes. Alternatively, use it as a dip (see the variation) or spread for tacos, burritos, raw or cooked vegetables, crackers, or chips.

1½ cups raw **cashews**, soaked in water for 1 hour and drained

1 orange or yellow **bell pepper**, diced

1 cup water

⅔ cup nutritional yeast flakes

4 large cloves **garlic**

Juice of 1 **lemon**

¾ teaspoon sweet **paprika**

¾ teaspoon sea salt

Put all the ingredients in a blender and process until smooth. Scrape down the blender jar and process for 15 seconds longer. Serve hot or cold. Stored in an airtight container in the refrigerator, the sauce will keep for 1 week.

SMOKY CASHEW CHEESE DIP: Decrease the amount of water to ⅓ cup. Replace the sweet paprika with ¾ teaspoon smoked paprika and ½ teaspoon chipotle chile powder or ancho chile powder.

SPICY NACHO CHEESE SAUCE: Replace the orange bell pepper with a red bell pepper. Replace the sweet paprika with 1 teaspoon chili powder, ½ teaspoon chipotle chile powder or cayenne, and ½ teaspoon ground cumin.

savory cashew GRAVY

Not only is this gravy meat-free and oil-free, but it's grain-free as well. It's thickened with a blend of cooked onions and garlic and pulverized cashews and chia seeds, all of which give it a delectably rich flavor. Use this gravy as a topping for baked tofu or tempeh, mashed potatoes, grains, or cooked vegetables.

3 cups low-sodium vegetable broth

⅓ cup finely diced yellow **onion** or **shallots**

1½ tablespoons minced **garlic**

½ cup raw **cashews**

2 tablespoons **chia seeds**

2 tablespoons nutritional yeast flakes

2 tablespoons reduced-sodium tamari

1½ teaspoons dried thyme

¼ teaspoon freshly ground **black pepper**

MAKES 2½ CUPS

Per ¼ cup:

53 calories

2 g protein

3 g fat (1 g sat)

3 g carbs

98 mg sodium

9 mg calcium

1 g fiber

Put ½ cup of the broth and the onion and garlic in a medium saucepan. Cook over medium heat, stirring occasionally, until the onion is soft and the broth has evaporated, about 5 minutes.

Put the cashews and chia seeds in a blender and process until finely ground. Scrape down the blender jar. Add the remaining 2½ cups of broth, the onion mixture, and the nutritional yeast, tamari, thyme, and pepper and process until smooth.

Transfer the mixture to the medium saucepan and cook over medium heat, whisking occasionally, until thickened, 3 to 5 minutes. Serve hot. Stored in an airtight container, the gravy will keep for 1 week in the refrigerator or 6 months in the freezer.

MUSHROOM-CASHEW GRAVY: When cooking the onion in the broth, add 2 cups (4 ounces) coarsely chopped button or crimini mushrooms. Do not process the mixture in the blender. Instead, stir the mushroom mixture into the gravy after it has thickened.

fermented foods, sauces, and spreads

chipotle-almond MAYO

MAKES 1 CUP

Per 2 tablespoons:

70 calories

0 g protein

7 g fat (1 g sat)

2 g carbs

124 mg sodium

28 mg calcium

0 g fiber

All you need is a blender and within minutes you can whip up a batch of this egg-free, dairy-free mayonnaise, which is enhanced with a smoky chipotle chile. Use it as a spread for sandwiches or as a sauce or dip for raw or cooked vegetables.

½ cup plain **almond milk**

2 tablespoons **lemon juice** or cider vinegar

1 tablespoon **ketchup**

1 canned chipotle **chile** in adobo sauce,
    or 1 teaspoon chipotle **chile powder**

½ teaspoon **garlic powder**

¼ teaspoon **onion powder**

¼ teaspoon sea salt

¼ cup **olive oil** or **avocado oil**

Put the milk, lemon juice, ketchup, chile, garlic powder, onion powder, and salt in a blender and process for 1 minute. Scrape down the blender jar. With the blender running, slowly add the oil through the opening in the lid and process for 1 minute.

Transfer to an airtight container. Refrigerate for at least 30 minutes before using to allow the mayo to thicken slightly. Stored in an airtight container in the refrigerator, the mayo will keep for 1 week.

> **HERB-ALMOND AIOLI:** Replace the ketchup and chipotle chile with ¾ cup fresh herbs (such as basil, cilantro, or parsley, or a combination), lightly packed, and replace the garlic powder with 2 large cloves garlic.

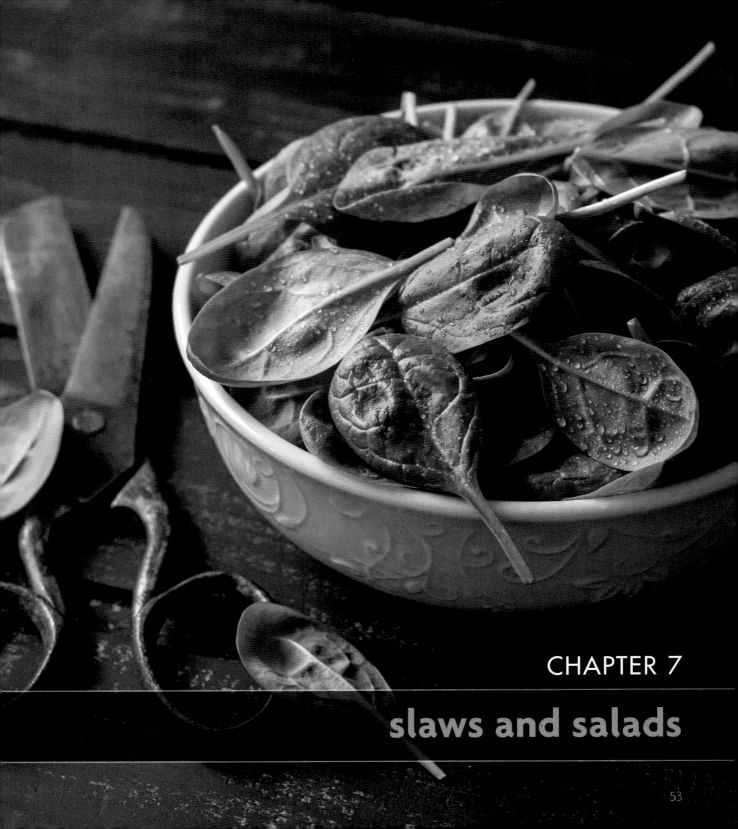

CHAPTER 7

slaws and salads

bavarian SLAW

MAKES 4 SERVINGS

Per serving:

100 calories

4 g protein

3 g fat (0.2 g sat)

18 g carbs

347 mg sodium

109 mg calcium

4 g fiber

Once maligned, Brussels sprouts have now become quite the rage. Their flavor complements their cruciferous cousins in this slaw, which is coated with a Bavarian-style sweet-and-sour dressing.

2 tablespoons maple syrup

2 tablespoons cider vinegar

2 tablespoons whole-grain or stone-ground **mustard**

½ teaspoon caraway seeds

½ teaspoon celery seeds

½ teaspoon sea salt

¼ teaspoon freshly ground **black pepper**

8 ounces **Brussels sprouts**, shredded

2 cups shredded **red cabbage**, lightly packed

1½ cups shredded **savoy or green cabbage**, lightly packed

1 cup shredded **carrots**, lightly packed

⅓ cup thinly sliced **green onions**

¼ cup chopped fresh **parsley**, lightly packed

1½ tablespoons poppy or **chia seeds**

To make the dressing, put the maple syrup, vinegar, mustard, caraway seeds, celery seeds, salt, and pepper in a small bowl and whisk to combine.

To make the slaw, put the Brussels sprouts, red cabbage, savoy cabbage, carrots, green onions, and parsley in a large bowl and toss gently to combine. Pour the dressing over the vegetable mixture. Sprinkle the poppy seeds over the top and toss gently until evenly distributed. Let sit for 10 minutes before serving to allow the Brussels sprouts and cabbage to wilt slightly.

> **TIP:** Use a food processor fitted with a thin slicing blade to quickly shred the Brussels sprouts. Note that shredded Brussels sprouts are sold in packages at many grocery stores; using them will make preparing this slaw even easier.

OMEGA kale slaw

Curly kale, shredded carrots and beets, and hemp and sesame seeds are coated in a creamy and slightly zesty tahini-based dressing. You'll easily get your daily dose of omega-3 and -6 fatty acids with just one helping of this slaw.

1 cup water

¼ cup tahini

3 tablespoons **lemon juice**

2 tablespoons **flaxseed oil** or **hemp seed oil**

1 tablespoon reduced-sodium tamari

2 teaspoons minced **garlic**

2 teaspoons peeled and grated fresh **ginger**

¼ teaspoon kelp powder

⅛ teaspoon **cayenne**

1 bunch (about 1 pound) **curly green or red kale**, stemmed and cut into thin strips

2 **carrots**, shredded

1 large **red beet**, peeled and shredded

1 large **gold beet**, peeled and shredded

⅓ cup thinly sliced **green onions**

¼ cup chopped fresh **parsley**, lightly packed, or 2 tablespoons chopped fresh dill

2 tablespoons **hemp seeds**

2 tablespoons sesame seeds

MAKES 4 SERVINGS

Per serving:

289 calories

9 g protein

21 g fat (1 g sat)

21 g carbs

204 mg sodium

231 mg calcium

7 g fiber

To make the dressing, put the water, tahini, lemon juice, oil, tamari, garlic, ginger, kelp powder, and cayenne in a blender and process until smooth.

To make the salad, put the kale, carrots, red beet, gold beet, green onions, and parsley in a large bowl and toss gently to combine. Pour the dressing over the vegetable mixture. Sprinkle the hemp seeds and sesame seeds over the top and toss gently until evenly distributed. Serve immediately.

shredded napa cabbage and vegetable SALAD

MAKES 6 SERVINGS

Per serving:

182 calories

5 g protein

14 g fat (2 g sat)

17 g carbs

215 mg sodium

55 mg calcium

2 g fiber

This Chinese-style salad features a mix of crisp napa and red cabbages, carrots, celery, daikon radish, snow peas, and mung bean sprouts, plus crunchy cashews and sesame seeds. Then everything is tossed together in a zesty lime and toasted sesame oil dressing.

4 cups shredded **napa cabbage**, lightly packed

1½ cups shredded **red cabbage**, lightly packed

1½ cups shredded **carrots**, lightly packed

1 cup thinly sliced **celery**, cut diagonally

1 cup mung bean sprouts, lightly packed

1 cup peeled and shredded **daikon radish**,
    or ½ cup thinly sliced **red radishes**

1 cup snap peas or pea pods, cut in half diagonally

⅓ cup thinly sliced **green onions**

⅓ cup fresh **cilantro**, lightly packed

2 tablespoons toasted sesame oil

2 tablespoons reduced-sodium tamari

Zest and juice of 1 **lime**

1½ tablespoons peeled and grated fresh **ginger**

1 tablespoon minced **garlic**

½ teaspoon crushed **red pepper** flakes (optional)

¼ teaspoon freshly ground **black pepper**

½ cup raw or roasted **cashew** pieces or roasted **peanuts**

2 tablespoons sesame seeds

Put the napa cabbage, red cabbage, carrots, celery, sprouts, daikon radish, snap peas, green onions, and cilantro in a large bowl and toss gently to combine.

To make the dressing, put the oil, tamari, lime zest and juice, ginger, garlic, optional red pepper flakes, and pepper in a small bowl and whisk to combine. Pour the dressing over the vegetable mixture. Sprinkle the cashews and sesame seeds over the top and toss gently until evenly distributed. Serve immediately.

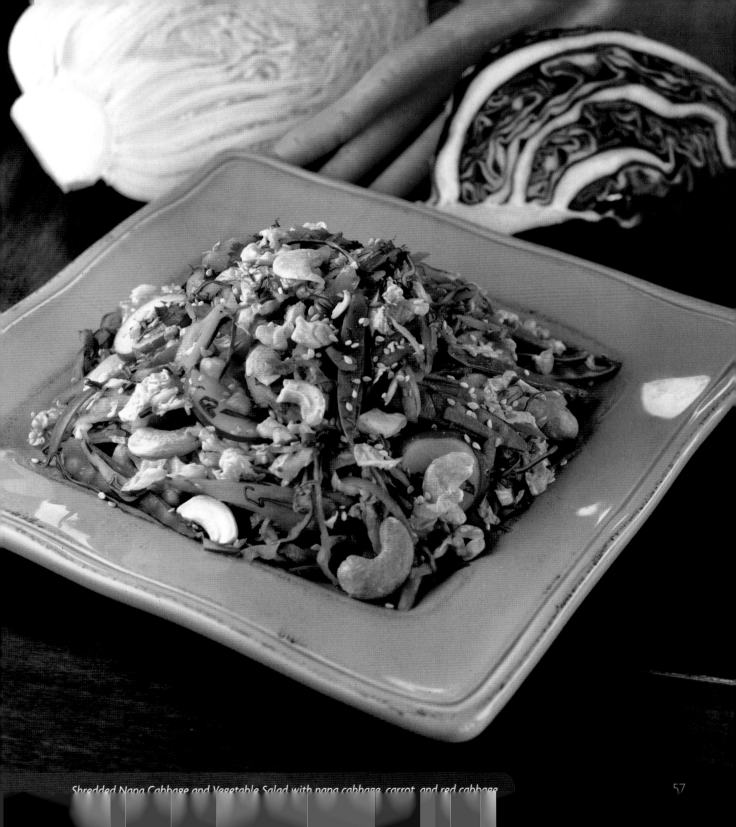

Shredded Napa Cabbage and Vegetable Salad with napa cabbage, carrot, and red cabbage

berrylicious spinach salad
WITH RASPBERRY CHIA-POPPY SEED DRESSING

MAKES 4 SERVINGS

Per serving:

155 calories

6 g protein

6 g fat (0.3 g sat)

21 g carbs

182 mg sodium

133 mg calcium

8 g fiber

Chia seeds, rather than oil, are used to thicken this fat-free raspberry dressing. It's speckled with poppy seeds, then drizzled over a fresh spinach and berry salad. Spring and summer, when fresh berries flood the market, are the ideal seasons for making this salad.

1 cup fresh **raspberries**

½ small red **onion**, thinly sliced into half-moons

½ cup water

2 tablespoons cider vinegar

1 tablespoon **chia seeds**

1 tablespoon agave nectar

¼ teaspoon dry **mustard**

¼ teaspoon sea salt

1½ teaspoons poppy seeds

6 cups baby **spinach**, lightly packed

1 cup fresh **blackberries** or **blueberries**

1 cup fresh **strawberries**, cut in half and thinly sliced

½ cup alfalfa sprouts, lightly packed

⅓ cup sliced **almonds**

To make the dressing, put ¼ cup of the raspberries, 1 tablespoon of the onion, and the water, vinegar, chia seeds, agave nectar, dry mustard, and salt in a blender and process for 1 minute. Transfer the dressing to a small bowl and stir in the poppy seeds.

To make the salad, put the spinach, remaining raspberries and onion, and the blackberries and strawberries in a large bowl and toss to combine. Scatter the sprouts and almonds over the top. Drizzle the dressing over each serving.

stone fruit, pecan, and pomegranate SALAD

To elevate the flavor of this salad, use a blend of mixed baby greens that includes arugula, as arugula's peppery undertones will add a pleasing complement to the sweet stone fruit, radicchio, watercress, and toasted pecans. The vinaigrette, made with tart pomegranate juice and nut oil, provides the perfect finishing touch.

⅔ cup **pomegranate juice**

2 tablespoons **orange** or **lemon juice**

1½ teaspoons Dijon **mustard**

3 tablespoons **walnut oil** or other nut oil

Sea salt

Freshly ground **black pepper**

4 cups mixed baby **greens**, lightly packed

1½ cups bite-sized torn pieces **radicchio**, lightly packed

1½ cups **watercress**, lightly packed

2 **nectarines** or **peaches**, thinly sliced

½ small red **onion**, thinly sliced into half-moons

¾ cup toasted pecan halves

½ cup **pomegranate seeds**

To make the dressing, put the pomegranate juice, orange juice, and mustard in a blender and process for 30 seconds. With the blender running, slowly add the oil through the opening in the lid and process for 1 minute. Season with salt and pepper to taste. Transfer to a small bowl.

To make the salad, put the baby greens, radicchio, and watercress in a large bowl and toss gently to combine. Add the nectarines, onion, pecans, and pomegranate seeds and toss gently until evenly distributed. Drizzle the dressing over each serving.

MAKES 4 SERVINGS

Per serving:

331 calories

6 g protein

24 g fat (2 g sat)

27 g carbs

101 mg sodium

107 mg calcium

53 g fiber

Note: Analysis doesn't include sea salt or freshly ground black pepper.

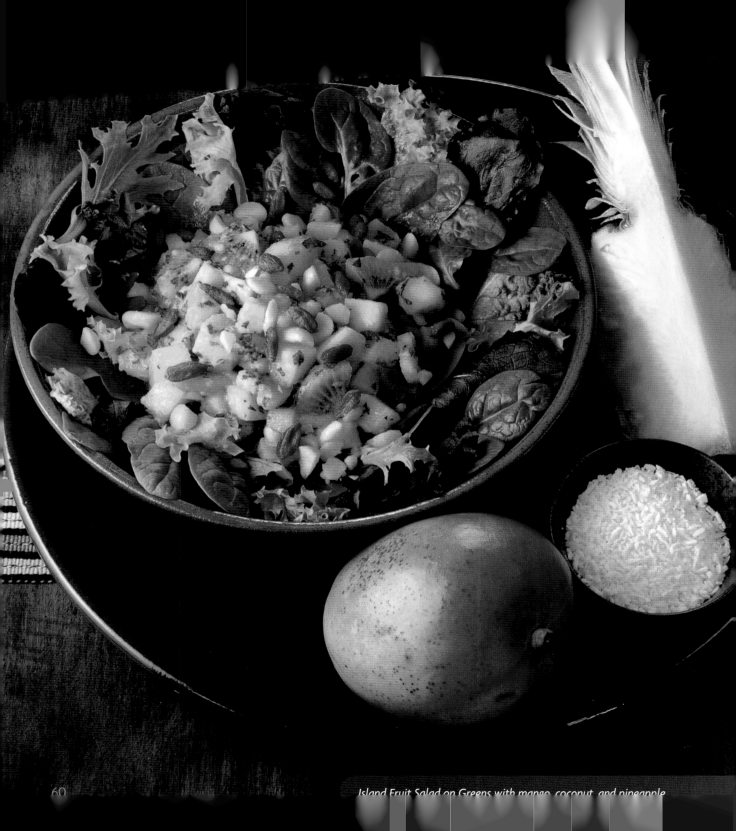

Island Fruit Salad on Greens with mango, coconut, and pineapple

island fruit salad ON GREENS

Tropical fruits are renowned for being succulent and sweet. For this salad, several varieties are briefly marinated in a vinaigrette made with pineapple juice and coconut oil to help marry their flavors before they're combined with leafy greens, macadamia nuts, coconut chips, and goji berries.

MAKES 4 SERVINGS

Per serving:

385 calories

4 g protein

26 g fat (13 g sat)

39 g carbs

33 mg sodium

43 mg calcium

6 g fiber

¼ cup **pineapple juice**

2 tablespoons **coconut oil**, melted

2 tablespoons agave nectar, or 2 tablespoons coconut sugar
  and 2 tablespoons water

2 tablespoons chopped fresh **mint** or **parsley**

1 tablespoon **lime juice**

1 tablespoon peeled and grated fresh **ginger**

½ teaspoon vanilla extract

1 cup peeled and diced fresh **papaya** or **mango** or frozen papaya
  or mango cubes, thawed

1 cup **pineapple** chunks or tidbits

1 **star fruit**, cut in half lengthwise and thinly sliced

1 **kiwi**, peeled, cut into quarters lengthwise, and thinly sliced

3 cups mixed baby **greens**, lightly packed

2 cups baby **spinach**, lightly packed

½ cup coarsely chopped raw or roasted **macadamia nuts**

⅓ cup unsweetened **coconut chips** or unsweetened shredded
  dried coconut

¼ cup **goji berries**, or ⅓ cup **pomegranate seeds**

Put the pineapple juice, oil, agave nectar, mint, lime juice, ginger, and vanilla extract in a medium bowl and whisk to combine. Add the papaya, pineapple, star fruit, and kiwi and stir to combine. Let marinate for 15 minutes.

Make a bed of the baby greens and spinach on a large platter. Arrange the fruit mixture on top of the greens. Scatter the macadamia nuts, coconut chips, and goji berries over the top. Serve immediately.

eat-the-rainbow salad
WITH CURRIED SESAME DRESSING

MAKES 6 SERVINGS

Per serving:

99 calories

3 g protein

8 g fat (1 g sat)

5 g carbs

82 mg sodium

38 mg calcium

2 g fiber

"Eat the rainbow" is a popular catchphrase for meals that contain a multicolored assortment of nutrient-rich fruits and veggies. Nearly every color of the rainbow is showcased in this salad, which is tossed with a curry-infused tahini dressing.

3 tablespoons water

2 tablespoons tahini

2 tablespoons **flaxseed oil**

1½ tablespoons cider vinegar

2 tablespoons chopped fresh **cilantro**

1 tablespoon minced **garlic**

1 teaspoon reduced-sodium tamari

½ teaspoon **curry powder**

¼ teaspoon ground **cumin**

3 large leaves rainbow **Swiss chard**, stemmed and cut into thin strips

2 large leaves curly red **kale**, stemmed and cut into thin strips

1 cup coarsely chopped **frisée** (curly endive) or **dandelion greens**, lightly packed

1 cup shredded red **cabbage**, lightly packed

2 stalks **celery**, thinly sliced

2 **carrots**, shredded

1 gold **beet**, peeled and shredded

1 **watermelon radish**, peeled and shredded

½ cup **red radishes**, cut in half and thinly sliced

To make the dressing, put the water, tahini, oil, vinegar, cilantro, garlic, tamari, curry powder, and cumin in a blender and process until smooth.

To make the salad, put the Swiss chard, kale, frisée, cabbage, celery, carrots, beet, watermelon radish, and red radishes in a large bowl and toss gently to combine. Pour the dressing over the top and toss gently until evenly distributed. Serve immediately.

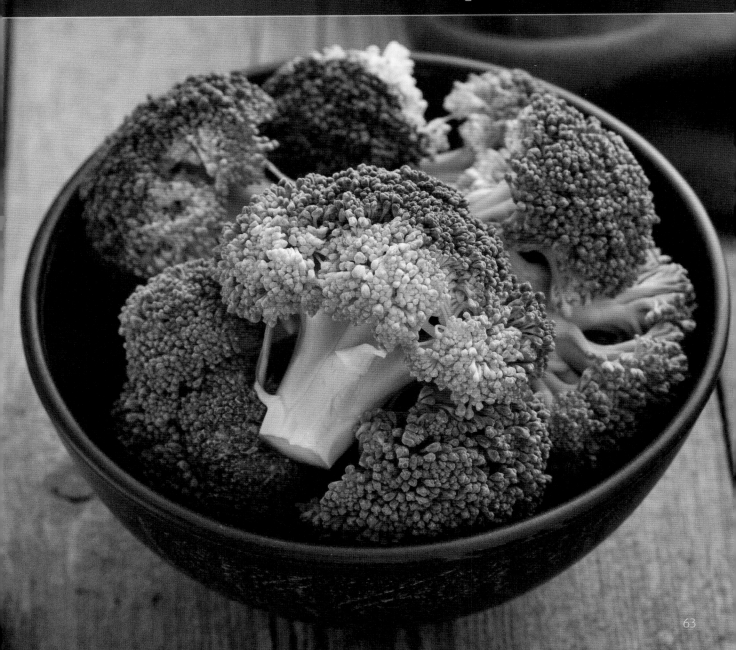

soups and stews

MISO vegetable soup

MAKES 4 SERVINGS

Per serving:

91 calories

6 g protein

3 g fat (1 g sat)

12 g carbs

526 mg sodium

72 mg calcium

4 g fiber

Depending on the type of miso you use, the broth of this soup will either have a mellow or rich flavor. This light yet filling vegetable soup can be prepared and enjoyed in under fifteen minutes, making it the ideal quick meal.

3 cups water

1 baby **bok choy**, cut into 1-inch strips

1 large **carrot**, cut in half lengthwise and thinly sliced diagonally

1 cup peeled and diced **daikon radish**

1 cup thinly sliced shiitake or other **mushrooms**

1 cup mung bean sprouts, lightly packed

⅔ cup fresh or frozen **edamame** or peas

½ cup thinly sliced **green onions**

1 tablespoon minced **garlic**

1 tablespoon peeled and grated fresh **ginger**

3 tablespoons miso

Raw or roasted sesame seeds

Wakame or nori flakes (optional)

Put the water, bok choy, carrot, daikon radish, mushrooms, sprouts, edamame, greens onions, garlic, and ginger in a large soup pot and stir to combine. Bring to a boil over high heat. Decrease the heat to low and simmer until the vegetables are tender, 8 to 10 minutes.

Put the miso and ½ cup of the soup broth in a small bowl and stir to combine. Add the miso mixture to the soup in the pot and stir to combine. Garnish with sesame seeds and wakame flakes if desired. Serve hot.

Note: Analysis doesn't include sesame seeds.

borscht

Borscht is a slightly tart and hearty soup that has sustained Eastern Europeans for generations, and rightfully so, as it contains many readily available ingredients from the region, including beets, cabbage, onion, and turnips. Serve portions plain or topped with a generous dollop of plain nondairy yogurt or vegan sour cream.

1 pound red **beets** with greens

3 cups low-sodium vegetable broth

2½ cups shredded green **cabbage**, lightly packed

1 large **turnip**, peeled and shredded

1 red or yellow **onion**, diced

1 **tomato**, diced

1 large **apple**, peeled, cored, and diced

¼ cup chopped fresh dill, or 1 tablespoon dried dill weed

2 tablespoons chopped fresh thyme, or 2 teaspoons dried thyme

1 bay leaf

¼ cup **orange juice**, or 2 tablespoons **lemon juice**

Sea salt

Freshly ground **black pepper**

Plain **nondairy yogurt** (preferably Greek-style) **or vegan sour cream** (optional)

MAKES 4 SERVINGS

Per serving:

101 calories

4 g protein

1 g fat (0.1 g sat)

23 g carbs

205 mg sodium

104 mg calcium

7 g fiber

Cut the greens from the beets and coarsely chop the stems and leaves. Peel and shred the beets. Put the beets, stems, and leaves in a large soup pot. Add the broth, cabbage, turnip, onion, tomato, apple, dill, thyme, and bay leaf and stir to combine. Bring to a boil over high heat. Cover, decrease the heat to low, and simmer until the vegetables are tender, 30 to 40 minutes.

Add the orange juice and stir to combine. Remove and discard the bay leaf. Season with salt and pepper to taste. Garnish each serving with a dollop of yogurt if desired. Serve hot.

> **TIP:** Greek-style yogurt has twice the protein of regular yogurt and much less sugar, which helps prevent insulin surges that can cause inflammation in the body. Greek-style nondairy yogurt and vegan sour cream can be found in the refrigerated case of most supermarkets and natural food stores.

Note: Analysis doesn't include sea salt or freshly ground black pepper.

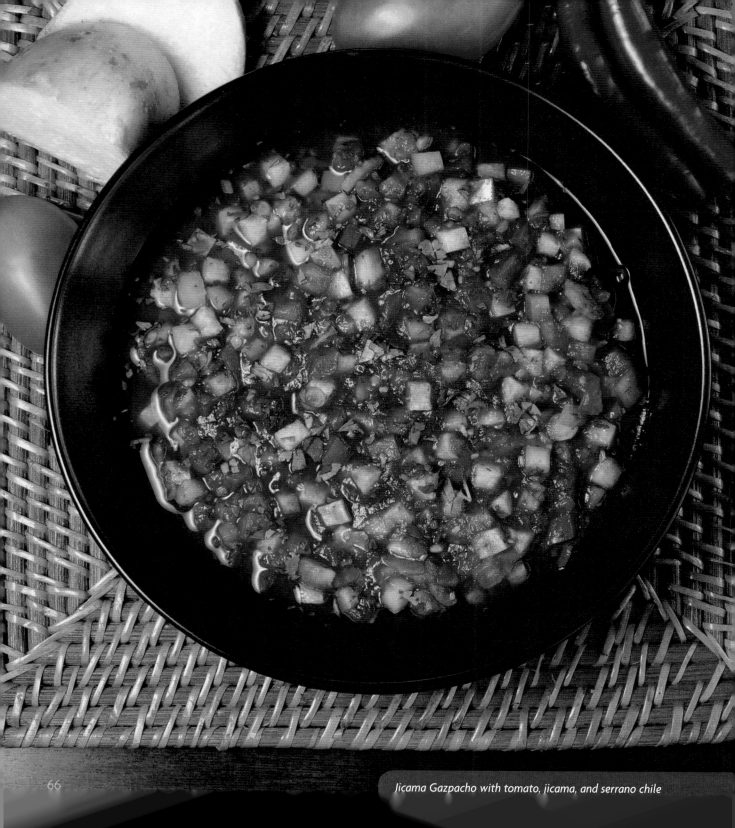

Jicama Gazpacho with tomato, jicama, and serrano chile

jicama GAZPACHO

Gazpacho is the quintessential midsummer soup and makes the most of the fresh vegetables and herbs commonly grown in gardens from coast to coast. This chunky, eye-catching version features tomatoes, celery, cucumber, bell pepper, and hot chile, as well as crisp jicama, all floating in a vinegar-enhanced tomato-based broth.

3 cups diced **tomatoes**

1½ cups peeled and diced **cucumber**

1½ cups peeled and diced **jicama**

1 red, orange, or yellow **bell pepper**, diced

⅔ cup thinly sliced **celery** (cut the stalk in half lengthwise before slicing)

½ cup thinly sliced **green onions**

1 serrano or jalapeño **chile**, seeded and finely diced (optional)

⅓ cup chopped fresh **cilantro**, lightly packed

⅓ cup chopped fresh **parsley**, lightly packed

1½ tablespoons minced **garlic**

½ teaspoon ground **cumin**

½ teaspoon crushed **red pepper** flakes (optional)

3 cups low-sodium **tomato juice** or **vegetable juice cocktail**

3 tablespoons balsamic or red wine vinegar

Sea salt

Freshly ground **black pepper**

Hot sauce (optional)

Put the tomatoes, cucumber, jicama, bell pepper, celery, green onions, optional chile, cilantro, parsley, garlic, cumin, and optional red pepper flakes in a large glass or ceramic bowl and stir to combine.

Add the tomato juice and vinegar and stir to combine. Season with salt and pepper to taste.

Cover and refrigerate for 1 hour or longer to let the flavors blend. Stir the soup again before serving. Serve cold, garnished with hot sauce if desired.

MAKES 4 SERVINGS

Per serving:

106 calories

3 g protein

1 g fat (0.1 g sat)

22 g carbs

153 mg sodium

64 mg calcium

6 g fiber

Note: Analysis doesn't include sea salt or freshly ground black pepper.

CREAMY broccoli and cauliflower SOUP

MAKES 4 SERVINGS

Per serving:

173 calories

8 g protein

7 g fat (1 g sat)

22 g carbs

90 mg sodium

179 mg calcium

8 g fiber

On a cold day, a thick and creamy soup fills the bill. The small amount of tahini adds luscious richness and elevates the flavor of the simmered broccoli and cauliflower from humdrum to yum!

3 cups low-sodium vegetable broth

3 cups small **broccoli** florets, or 1 package (16 ounces) **frozen broccoli florets**

3 cups small **cauliflower** florets, or 1 package (16 ounces) **frozen cauliflower florets**

1 **rutabaga**, peeled and finely diced

1 **leek**, cut in half lengthwise and thinly sliced

2 tablespoons minced **garlic**

2 teaspoons dried tarragon

1 teaspoon dried thyme

1 bay leaf

1 cup plain nondairy milk

3 tablespoons tahini

2 tablespoon nutritional yeast flakes

¼ cup chopped fresh **parsley**, lightly packed

Sea salt

Freshly ground **black** or **white pepper**

Put the broth, broccoli, cauliflower, rutabaga, leek, garlic, tarragon, thyme, and bay leaf in a large soup pot. Bring to a boil over high heat. Cover, decrease the heat to low, and simmer until the vegetables are tender, 25 to 30 minutes. Remove and discard the bay leaf.

Transfer 2 cups of the soup to a blender. Add the milk, tahini, and nutritional yeast and process until smooth. Pour into the soup in the pot, add the parsley, and stir to combine. Season with salt and pepper to taste. Serve hot.

Note: Analysis doesn't include sea salt or freshly ground black or white pepper.

SMOKY pumpkin-chipotle SOUP

Using pumpkin purée in this soup rather than freshly roasted pumpkin quickly achieves a creamy base. The soup's smoky flavor comes from chipotle chiles in adobo sauce, which can be found in cans in the international section of most supermarkets.

MAKES 4 SERVINGS

Per serving:

164 calories

4 g protein

7 g fat (1 g sat)

20 g carbs

780 mg sodium

122 mg calcium

5 g fiber

1 cup diced **shallots**, or 1½ cups diced yellow **onions**

1 tablespoon **olive oil**

2 tablespoons minced **garlic**

1 cup plain nondairy milk

2 canned chipotle **chiles** in adobo sauce (see tip)

1½ tablespoons arrowroot or cornstarch

1 tablespoon reduced-sodium tamari

1 teaspoon ground **cumin**

1 teaspoon sea salt

3 cups low-sodium vegetable broth

1 can (15 ounces) **pumpkin** purée

Plain nondairy yogurt (preferably Greek-style) or vegan sour cream (optional)

Put the shallots and oil in a large soup pot and cook over medium-high heat, stirring occasionally, for 5 minutes. Add the garlic and cook, stirring occasionally, until the shallots are soft and lightly browned, about 5 minutes.

Transfer to a blender. Add the milk, chiles, arrowroot, tamari, cumin, and salt and process until smooth. Scrape down the blender jar and process for 15 seconds longer.

Transfer to a large soup pot. Add the broth and pumpkin purée and stir to combine. Cook over medium-high heat, stirring occasionally, until the soup is hot and bubbling, 6 to 8 minutes. Garnish each serving with a dollop of yogurt if desired. Serve hot.

> **TIP:** If you can't find canned chipotle chiles in adobo sauce, replace them with 2 teaspoons chipotle chile powder, or 1 teaspoon smoked paprika and 1 teaspoon cayenne or ancho chile powder.

mexicali veggie CHILI

MAKES 6 SERVINGS

Per serving:

278 calories

14 g protein

6 g fat (1 g sat)

47 g carbs

610 mg sodium

117 mg calcium

15 g fiber

A big pot of chili makes for a super supper during the fall and winter months. This thick and hearty chili is packed with a colorful assortment of diced vegetables, crushed tomatoes, two kinds of beans, and cacao powder, which, surprisingly, deepens the flavor of the chili.

1 red or yellow **onion**, diced

1 red, orange, or yellow **bell pepper**, diced

1 **sweet potato**, peeled and diced

1 small **zucchini**, diced

1 small **yellow squash**, diced

1½ tablespoons **olive oil**

1 serrano or jalapeño **chile**, seeded and finely diced (optional)

2 tablespoons minced **garlic**

1½ teaspoons **chili powder**

1½ teaspoons dried **oregano**

1 teaspoon ground **cumin**

¼ teaspoon **cayenne** or chipotle **chile powder** (optional)

1 can (28 ounces) crushed **tomatoes**

1 can (15 ounces) black beans, drained and rinsed

1 can (15 ounces) kidney beans, drained and rinsed

1½ cups water

1 tablespoon **cacao powder** or unsweetened cocoa powder

⅓ cup chopped fresh **cilantro**, lightly packed

Sea salt

Freshly ground **black pepper**

1 Hass **avocado**, diced

Hot sauce (optional)

Put the onion, bell pepper, sweet potato, zucchini, yellow squash, and oil in a large soup pot and cook, stirring occasionally, for 10 minutes. Add the chile, garlic, chili powder, oregano, cumin, and optional cayenne and cook, stirring occasionally, for 2 minutes.

Note: Analysis doesn't include sea salt or freshly ground black pepper.

Add the tomatoes, black beans, kidney beans, water, and cacao powder and stir to combine. Bring to a boil over high heat. Cover, decrease the heat to low, and simmer, stirring occasionally, until the vegetables are tender, about 30 minutes. Add the cilantro and stir until evenly distributed. Season with salt and pepper to taste. Garnish each serving with some of the avocado and a little hot sauce if desired. Serve hot.

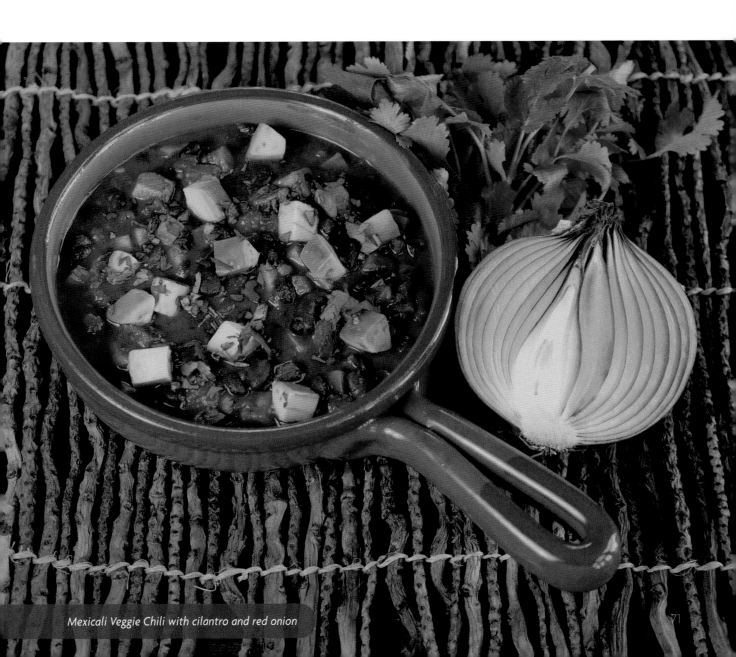

Mexicali Veggie Chili with cilantro and red onion

white bean and swiss chard SOUP

MAKES 6 SERVINGS

Per serving:

198 calories

14 g protein

3 g fat (0.1 g sat)

32 g carbs

198 mg sodium

59 mg calcium

13 g fiber

Although using dried beans rather than canned lengthens the preparation time of this soup, it creates the most delectable broth. Feel free to use either green, red, or rainbow Swiss chard, as all these varieties pair well with white beans.

3 quarts water

1½ cups dried white beans (such as cannellini or great Northern), sorted and rinsed

1 bay leaf

1½ cups diced **celery**

1½ cups diced yellow **onions**

1 tablespoon **olive oil**

2 tablespoons minced **garlic**

1½ teaspoons dried rosemary

1 teaspoon dried **basil**

1 teaspoon dried marjoram or **oregano**

½ teaspoon rubbed sage

½ teaspoon crushed **red pepper** flakes (optional)

1 bunch (about 1 pound) **Swiss chard**, stems and leaves coarsely chopped

2 tablespoons nutritional yeast flakes

Sea salt

Freshly ground **black pepper**

Put the water, beans, and bay leaf in a large soup pot and bring to a boil over high heat. Cover, decrease the heat to low, and simmer for 1 hour.

While the beans are cooking, put the celery, onions, and oil in a large cast-iron or nonstick skillet and cook over medium-high heat, stirring occasionally, for 10 minutes. Add the garlic, rosemary, basil, marjoram, sage, and optional red pepper flakes and cook, stirring occasionally, for 2 minutes.

Add the vegetable mixture and Swiss chard to the soup pot, stir to combine, and simmer until the beans are soft, about 30 minutes. Remove and discard the bay leaf. Add the nutritional yeast and stir until well incorporated. Season with salt and pepper to taste. Serve hot.

Note: Analysis doesn't include sea salt or freshly ground black pepper.

ROASTED winter squash, lentil, and kale STEW

Cubes of winter squash are tossed with olive oil, cumin, and turmeric and then roasted to perfection in the oven. Sure, you could just throw the raw cubes into the simmering lentil mixture, but this added step really amplifies the final flavor of this hearty stew.

1 large (about 3 pounds) **winter squash** (such as butternut, buttercup, kabocha, or red kuri), **peeled, seeded, and cut into 1-inch cubes**

1 tablespoon **olive oil**

1 teaspoon ground **cumin**

1 teaspoon ground **turmeric** or **curry powder**

6 cups water

1½ cups dried brown lentils, sorted and rinsed

1 yellow **onion**, diced

2 stalks **celery**, thinly sliced

1½ tablespoons minced **garlic**

1½ tablespoons peeled and grated fresh **ginger**

1 teaspoon dried **basil**

1 teaspoon dried thyme

1 bunch (about 1 pound) curly or lacinato **kale**, stemmed and cut into thin strips

2 tablespoons nutritional yeast flakes

Sea salt

Freshly ground **black pepper**

MAKES 6 SERVINGS

Per serving:

346 calories

20 g protein

4 g fat (1 g sat)

66 g carbs

55 mg sodium

263 mg calcium

23 g fiber

Preheat the oven to 400 degrees F. Line a baking sheet with parchment paper or a silicone baking mat. Put the squash, oil, cumin, and turmeric in a large bowl and stir to evenly coat the squash. Transfer to the lined baking sheet. Bake for 20 to 25 minutes, until the squash cubes are tender and lightly browned around the edges. Remove from the oven and set aside.

Put the water, lentils, onion, celery, garlic, ginger, basil, and thyme in a large soup pot and stir to combine. Bring to a boil over high heat. Cover, decrease the heat to low, and simmer for 30 minutes.

Add the roasted squash, kale, and nutritional yeast and stir to combine. Simmer until the lentils and kale are tender, about 10 minutes. Season with salt and pepper to taste. Serve hot.

ROASTED WINTER SQUASH, RED LENTIL, AND KALE STEW: Decrease the water to 4 cups and replace the brown lentils with 1½ cups dried red lentils. Decrease the lentil cooking time to 15 minutes.

Note: Analysis doesn't include sea salt or freshly ground black pepper.

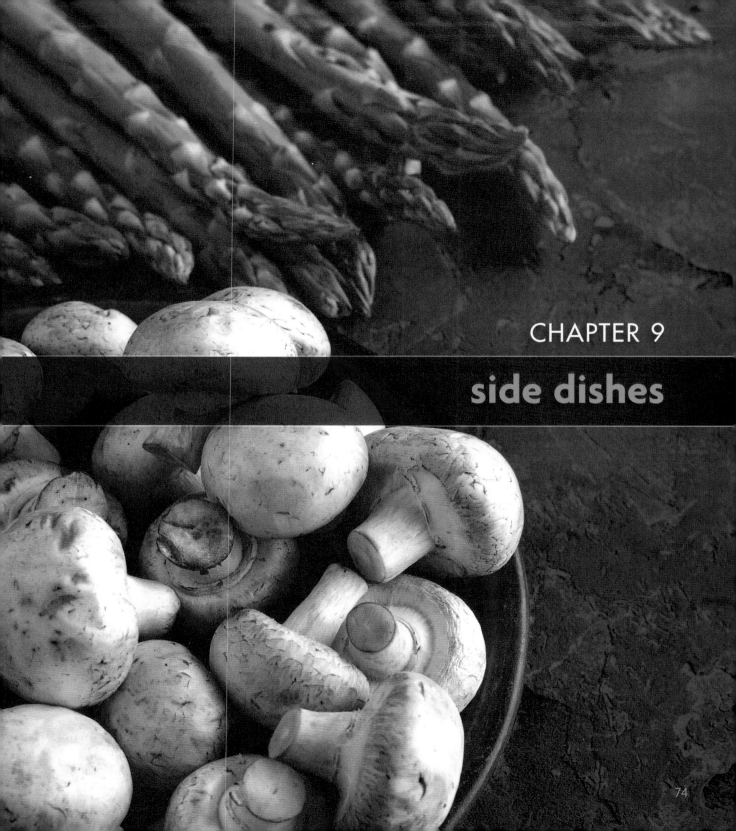

CHAPTER 9

side dishes

74

mushroom, asparagus, and ancient grains MEDLEY

Amaranth, millet, and quinoa are ancient grains packed with protein, fiber, and B vitamins. Even though their seed kernels are different sizes, they cook in roughly the same amount of time. This medley, featuring asparagus and mushrooms in combination with these three grains, can be ready in under thirty minutes.

½ cup amaranth

½ cup millet

½ cup quinoa

2¼ cups low-sodium vegetable broth or water

8 ounces crimini or button **mushrooms**, cut in half and thinly sliced

1 cup diced **shallots** or yellow **onion**

1 tablespoon **olive oil**

8 ounces fresh asparagus, cut into 1-inch pieces, or 1 package (9 ounces) frozen cut asparagus

1½ tablespoons minced **garlic**

1 teaspoon dried **basil**

1 teaspoon dried **oregano** or marjoram

1 tablespoon nutritional yeast flakes

1 tablespoon reduced-sodium tamari

Sea salt

Freshly ground **black pepper**

MAKES 6 SERVINGS

Per serving:

198 calories

8 g protein

3 g fat (0.3 g sat)

36 g carbs

88 mg sodium

59 mg calcium

5 g fiber

Put the amaranth, millet, and quinoa in a fine-mesh strainer and rinse under running water. Put the grains and broth in a medium saucepan and bring to a boil over high heat. Cover, decrease the heat to low, and simmer until the grains are tender and all the broth is absorbed, 18 to 20 minutes. Remove from the heat.

While the grains are cooking, put the mushrooms, shallots, and oil in a large cast-iron or nonstick skillet and cook over medium-high heat, stirring occasionally, for 5 minutes. Add the asparagus, garlic, basil, and oregano and cook, stirring occasionally, until the vegetables are tender, about 5 minutes.

Fluff the grains with a fork to separate. Add the grains, nutritional yeast, and tamari to the vegetable mixture and stir until evenly distributed. Season with salt and pepper to taste. Serve hot.

Note: Analysis doesn't include sea salt or freshly ground black pepper.

MEXICAN-STYLE gold beet "rice"

MAKES 4 SERVINGS

Per serving:

192 calories

6 g protein

6 g fat (1 g sat)

31 g carbs

167 mg sodium

65 mg calcium

8 g fiber

Going grain-free? No problem! In minutes, with the help of a food processor, you can cleverly transform cubes of gold beets into vegetable "rice." The golden bits add a touch of sweetness to this modernized version of Mexican rice, which is topped with diced avocado.

1½ pounds gold **beets**, peeled and cut into 1-inch cubes

1 cup diced yellow **onion**

1 serrano or jalapeño **chile**, seeded and finely diced (optional)

1½ tablespoons olive oil

1 package (10 ounces) **frozen mixed vegetables** (**carrots**, corn, and peas)

¾ cup diced **tomatoes**

1 tablespoon minced **garlic**

1 tablespoon **chili powder**

⅓ cup thinly sliced **green onions**

⅓ cup chopped fresh **cilantro**, lightly packed

Sea salt

Freshly ground **black pepper**

1 Hass **avocado**, diced

Put the beets in a food processor and pulse into rice-sized pieces. Transfer to a large cast-iron or nonstick skillet and add the onion, optional chile, and oil. Cook over medium-high heat, stirring occasionally, for 5 minutes.

Add the mixed vegetables, tomatoes, garlic, and chili powder and cook, stirring occasionally, until the vegetables are tender, about 5 minutes. Add the green onions and cilantro and stir until evenly distributed. Season with salt and pepper to taste. Garnish each serving with some of the avocado. Serve hot.

VARIATION: Replace the gold beets with 1½ pounds sweet potatoes, peeled and cut into 1-inch cubes.

Note: Analysis doesn't include sea salt or freshly ground black pepper.

cauliflower fried "rice"
WITH PINEAPPLE AND CASHEWS

With just a standard box grater, a head of cauliflower can be easily transformed into grain-free vegetable "rice." In this recipe, cauliflower rice is cooked with a colorful combination of diced vegetables, fresh garlic and ginger, sweet pineapple, and crunchy cashews. The flavor rivals traditional fried rice.

1 head (1½ pounds) **cauliflower**

⅔ cup finely diced **carrot**

⅔ cup finely diced **celery**

⅔ cup finely diced red **bell pepper**

2 tablespoons toasted sesame oil

2 cups shredded green **cabbage**, lightly packed

1½ tablespoons minced **garlic**

1½ tablespoons peeled and grated fresh **ginger**

1 cup fresh or frozen **pineapple** chunks or tidbits

¼ cup thinly sliced **green onions**

2 tablespoons reduced-sodium tamari

¾ teaspoon crushed **red pepper** flakes (optional)

½ teaspoon freshly ground **black pepper**

⅔ cup roasted **cashew** pieces

Grate the cauliflower with a box grater. Transfer to a large bowl.

Put the carrot, celery, bell pepper, and oil in a large cast-iron or nonstick skillet and cook over medium-high heat, stirring occasionally, for 5 minutes. Add the cauliflower, cabbage, garlic, and ginger and cook, stirring occasionally, until the vegetables are tender, about 5 minutes.

Add the pineapple, green onions, tamari, optional red pepper flakes, and pepper and cook, stirring occasionally, for 2 minutes. Add the cashews and stir until evenly distributed. Serve hot.

MAKES 4 SERVINGS

Per serving:

269 calories

8 g protein

16 g fat (3 g sat)

28 g carbs

400 mg sodium

86 mg calcium

7 g fiber

side dishes

FESTIVE wild rice

MAKES 4 SERVINGS

Per serving:

387 calories

7 g protein

15 g fat (1 g sat)

57 g carbs

667 mg sodium

50 mg calcium

5 g fiber

Not only is wild rice not related to rice, but it's also not even a grain. It's actually the grain-like seed of a marsh grass that was first harvested by Native Americans. Nutty-tasting wild rice combines deliciously with the toasted pecans, savory vegetables, sweet potato, and dried fruits in this dish.

4 cups low-sodium vegetable broth or water

1¼ cups wild rice, rinsed

1 **sweet potato**, peeled and cut into ½-inch cubes

1½ tablespoons toasted sesame oil

1 cup thinly sliced **celery**

½ cup thinly sliced **green onions**

⅓ cup dried **cherries**, or ¼ cup dried **cranberries**

1½ tablespoons peeled and grated fresh **ginger**

2 teaspoons dried thyme

½ cup chopped fresh **parsley**, lightly packed

½ cup toasted pecan halves or chopped pieces

1 tablespoon reduced-sodium tamari

Sea salt

Freshly ground **black pepper**

Put the broth and wild rice in a medium saucepan and bring to a boil over high heat. Cover, decrease the heat to low, and simmer until the wild rice is tender and all the water is absorbed, 45 to 50 minutes. Remove from the heat.

While the wild rice is cooking, put the sweet potatoes and oil in a large cast-iron or nonstick skillet and cook over medium-high heat, stirring occasionally, for 5 minutes. Add the celery and cook, stirring occasionally, for 3 minutes. Add the green onions, dried cherries, ginger, and thyme and cook, stirring occasionally, until the vegetables are tender, 2 to 3 minutes. Remove from the heat.

Fluff the wild rice with a fork to separate. Add the wild rice, parsley, pecans, and tamari to the vegetable mixture and stir until evenly distributed. Season with salt and pepper to taste. Serve hot or at room temperature.

Note: Analysis doesn't include sea salt or freshly ground black pepper.

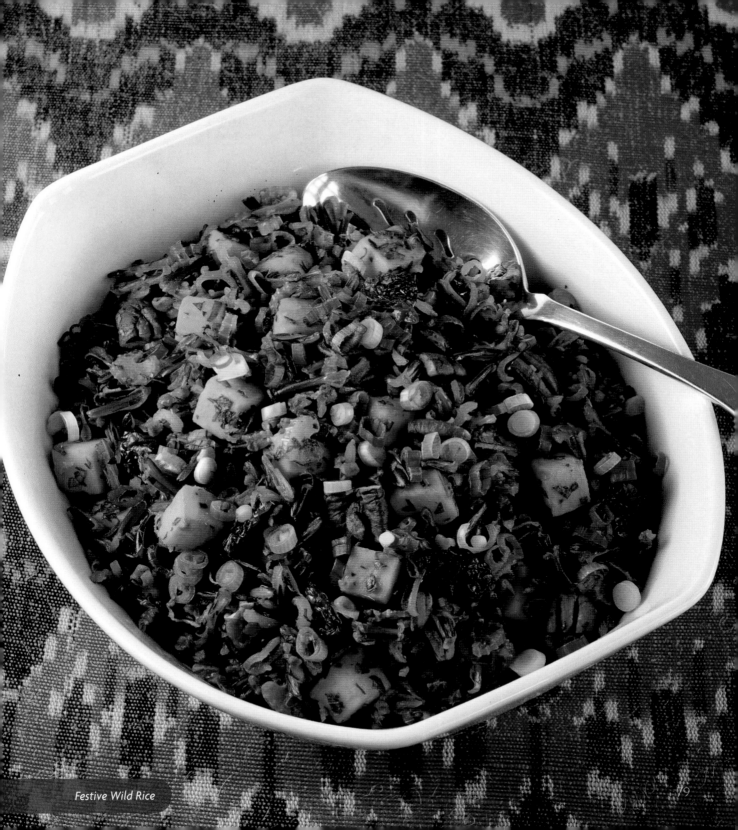

Festive Wild Rice

mujadara

MAKES 6 SERVINGS

Per serving:

273 calories

12 g protein

5 g fat (1 g sat)

47 g carbs

7 mg sodium

40 mg calcium

12 g fiber

Mujadara is a Middle Eastern lentil and rice dish that's flavored with aromatic spices and typically topped with savory caramelized onions. If you're looking for an easy, inexpensive side dish, give this recipe a try. To serve it the traditional way, top each serving with a dollop of nondairy yogurt.

½ large yellow **onion**, diced

1½ tablespoons sunflower oil or canola oil

4 cups water

1 cup dried brown lentils, sorted and rinsed

1 cup long-grain brown rice

1 teaspoon ground **coriander**

1 teaspoon ground **cumin**

½ teaspoon allspice

½ teaspoon ground **cinnamon**

1½ large yellow **onions**, thinly sliced

Sea salt

Freshly ground **black pepper**

Plain nondairy **yogurt** (preferably Greek-style; optional)

Put the diced onion and ½ tablespoon of the oil in a large saucepan and cook over medium-high heat, stirring occasionally, until the onion is soft and lightly browned, 6 to 8 minutes.

Add the water, lentils, rice, coriander, cumin, allspice, and cinnamon and stir to combine. Bring to a boil over high heat. Cover, decrease the heat to low, and simmer until the lentils and rice are tender and all the water is absorbed, 35 to 45 minutes. Remove from the heat.

While the lentils are cooking, make the caramelized onions. Put the sliced onions and the remaining tablespoon of oil in a large cast-iron or nonstick skillet. Cook over medium-high heat, stirring occasionally, for 5 minutes. Sprinkle with a pinch of salt. Decrease the heat to low and cook, stirring occasionally, until the onions are soft and golden brown, 30 to 35 minutes. For crispier onions, cook for 45 to 55 minutes.

Note: Analysis doesn't include sea salt or freshly ground black pepper.

Season the lentil mixture with salt and pepper to taste. Transfer to a large bowl or platter. Top with the caramelized onions. Garnish each serving with a dollop of yogurt if desired. Serve hot.

MAYAN black beans

Beans, corn, and squash were staple crops of the ancient Mayans of Mexico. For this marinated side dish, they're paired with cherry tomatoes and cilantro, tossed with a spicy marinade, and topped with avocado and pumpkin seeds.

2 tablespoons **avocado oil** or other oil

Zest and juice of 1 **lime**

¾ teaspoon **chili powder**

¾ teaspoon dried **oregano**

1 can (15 ounces) **black beans**, drained and rinsed

1 cup fresh or frozen **corn** kernels, thawed

1 cup halved cherry **tomatoes**

1 cup diced **zucchini**

⅓ cup chopped fresh **cilantro**, lightly packed

1 serrano or jalapeño **chile**, seeded and finely diced (optional)

Sea salt

Freshly ground **black pepper**

1 Hass **avocado**, diced

⅓ cup raw or roasted **pumpkin seeds**

Put the oil, lime zest and juice, chili powder, and oregano in a large bowl and whisk to combine. Add the beans, corn, tomatoes, zucchini, cilantro, and optional chile and stir to combine. Season with salt and pepper to taste. Scatter the avocado and pumpkin seeds over the top. Serve immediately.

MAKES 4 SERVINGS

Per serving:

328 calories

13 g protein

20 g fat (3 g sat)

34 g carbs

465 mg sodium

46 mg calcium

11 g fiber

Note: Analysis doesn't include sea salt or freshly ground black pepper.

white beans WITH ESCAROLE

MAKES 4 SERVINGS

Per serving:

160 calories

9 g protein

4 g fat (0 g sat)

25 g carbs

332 mg sodium

106 mg calcium

12 g fiber

Escarole is a variety of endive that has broad leaves with ragged edges and a slightly bitter flavor that works well in salads, soups, and side dishes. It's a common ingredient in Italian cuisine and is often paired with white beans, which was the inspiration for this tasty combination.

1 cup diced yellow **onion**

1 tablespoon **olive oil**

1 large head (1½ to 2 pounds) **escarole**, cut into 1-inch strips

2 tablespoons minced **garlic**

1 teaspoon dried **basil**

1 teaspoon dried **oregano**

½ teaspoon crushed **red pepper** flakes

1 can (15 ounces) **white beans** (such as cannellini, great Northern, or white kidney), **drained and rinsed**

1½ cups low-sodium vegetable broth or water

1 tablespoon nutritional yeast flakes

Sea salt

Freshly ground **black pepper**

Put the onion and oil in a large cast-iron or nonstick skillet and cook over medium-high heat, stirring occasionally, for 5 minutes. Add the escarole, garlic, basil, oregano, and red pepper flakes and cook, stirring occasionally, until the escarole has wilted, about 5 minutes.

Add the beans, broth, and nutritional yeast and stir to combine. Decrease the heat to low and simmer until the escarole is tender and all the water is absorbed, about 15 minutes. Season with salt and pepper to taste. Serve hot.

Note: Analysis doesn't include sea salt or freshly ground black pepper.

green and yellow beans AMANDINE

Steam-frying is a great way to cook vegetables until they're crisp-tender. Fresh ginger and garlic add zest, while toasted sesame oil provides a bit of smokiness to this side dish, which is topped with crunchy toasted almonds.

⅔ cup sliced **almonds**

8 ounces fresh green beans, cut in half, or 1 package (10 ounces) **frozen cut green beans**

8 ounces fresh yellow wax beans, cut in half, or 1 package (10 ounces) **frozen cut yellow wax beans**

½ cup low-sodium vegetable broth or water

1½ tablespoons minced **garlic**

1½ tablespoons peeled and grated fresh **ginger**

½ teaspoon crushed **red pepper** flakes

½ teaspoon freshly ground **black pepper**

¼ cup chopped fresh **parsley**, lightly packed

1 tablespoon reduced-sodium tamari

1 tablespoon toasted sesame oil

Put the almonds in a large cast-iron or nonstick skillet and cook over medium heat, stirring occasionally, until the almonds are lightly toasted and fragrant, 3 to 5 minutes. Transfer to a small plate.

Put the green beans, yellow wax beans, broth, garlic, ginger, red pepper flakes, and pepper in the skillet and cook over medium heat, stirring occasionally, until the green beans and yellow wax beans are crisp-tender, 6 to 8 minutes. Add the parsley, tamari, and oil and stir until evenly distributed. Remove from the heat. Sprinkle the almonds over the top. Serve hot.

MAKES 4 SERVINGS

Per serving:

206 calories

8 g protein

14 g fat (1 g sat)

14 g carbs

138 mg sodium

116 mg calcium

7 g fiber

Note: Analysis doesn't include sea salt or freshly ground black pepper.

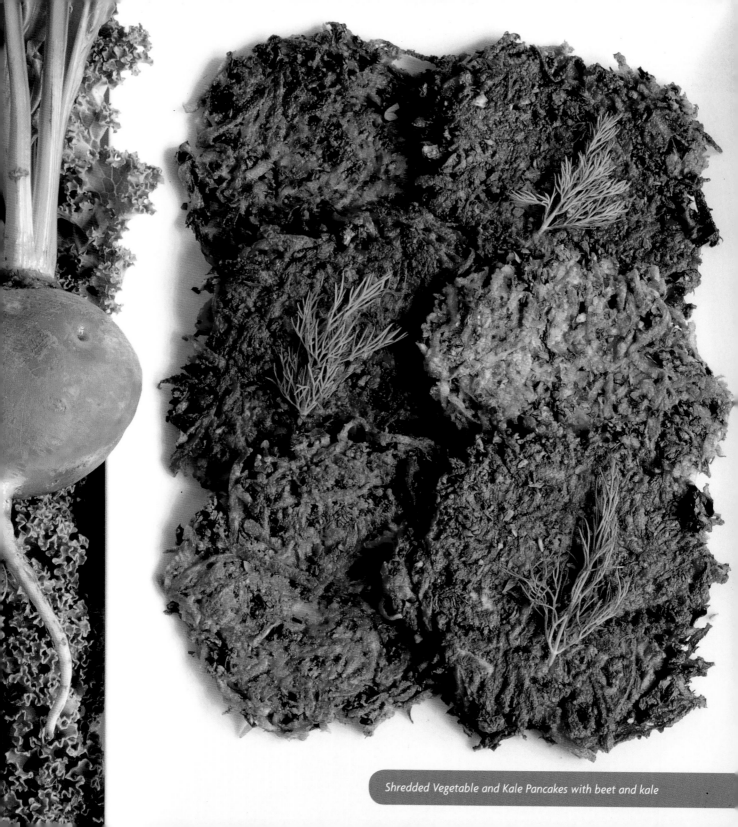

Shredded Vegetable and Kale Pancakes with beet and kale

shredded vegetable and kale PANCAKES

Expand your potato-pancake repertoire by replacing the spuds with other root vegetables. These crisp pancakes are made with shredded beets, carrots, and turnips, along
with some chopped kale, chives, and fresh herbs for added flavor and visual appeal.
Serve them plain or topped with nondairy yogurt, vegan sour cream, or applesauce.

MAKES 12 PANCAKES

Per pancake:

65 calories

2 g protein

2 g fat (0.2 g sat)

9 g carbs

217 mg sodium

28 mg calcium

2 g fiber

¾ cup steel-cut oats

1 large (8 ounces) **turnip**, peeled and shredded

1 large (8 ounces) gold or red **beet**, peeled and shredded

2 large **carrots**, peeled and shredded

1 cup stemmed and coarsely chopped **kale**, lightly packed

¼ cup chopped fresh **parsley**, lightly packed

2 tablespoons finely chopped **chives**

2 tablespoons chopped fresh dill, or 2 teaspoons dried dill weed

2 tablespoons nutritional yeast flakes

1 teaspoon **garlic powder**

1 teaspoon sea salt

½ teaspoon freshly ground **black pepper**

1½ tablespoons canola or other oil

Put the oats in a blender and process into a fine flour, about 30 seconds. Set aside.

Put a colander in the sink. Put the turnip, beet, and carrots in the colander and squeeze with your hands to remove excess moisture. Transfer to a
large bowl. Add the kale, parsley, chives, dill, nutritional yeast, garlic powder,
salt, and pepper and stir to combine. Add the reserved oat flour and stir until
evenly distributed.

Cook the pancakes in three batches. Put ½ tablespoon of the oil in a large
cast-iron or nonstick skillet and heat over medium-high heat. When the skillet is hot, portion the vegetable mixture into it, using ¼ cup for each pancake.
Slightly flatten each pancake with a spatula.

Cook until the pancakes are golden brown and crispy on the bottom,
3 to 5 minutes. Flip with a spatula and cook until the other side is brown
and crispy, 3 to 5 minutes longer. Repeat the process with the remaining oil
and vegetable mixture. Serve immediately.

squash and cherry tomato medley
WITH OLIVES

The flavors and textures of summer squash, zucchini, and cherry tomatoes complement each other beautifully. This colorful combination is further enhanced with the addition of salty olives and fresh herbs.

2 **yellow squashes**, cut in half lengthwise and sliced into ½-inch-thick half-moons

2 **zucchini**, cut in half lengthwise and sliced into ½-inch-thick half-moons

1 tablespoon **olive oil**

3 cups cherry **tomatoes**

½ cup pitted green or black **olives** or a combination, cut in half

2 tablespoons minced **garlic**

⅓ cup chopped fresh **basil**, lightly packed

2 tablespoons chopped fresh marjoram or **oregano**, or 2 teaspoons dried

1½ tablespoons nutritional yeast flakes

Sea salt

Freshly ground **black pepper**

Put the yellow squashes, zucchini, and oil in a large cast-iron or nonstick skillet and cook over medium-high heat, stirring occasionally, for 5 minutes. Add the tomatoes, olives, and garlic and cook, stirring occasionally, until the yellow squashes and zucchini are crisp-tender and the tomatoes are just starting to soften and release their juices, about 3 minutes.

Add the basil, marjoram, and nutritional yeast and stir until evenly distributed. Season with salt and pepper to taste. Serve hot.

> **VARIATION:** Replace the cherry tomatoes with 2 large heirloom tomatoes, cut into 2-inch chunks (about 3 cups).

Note: Analysis doesn't include sea salt or freshly ground black pepper.

WHIPPED root vegetables

Move over mashed potatoes—this luscious, creamy purée of celery root, rutabaga, and turnips is poised to take your place! It's especially welcome during the fall and winter holidays and is a great way to work these under-appreciated vegetables into meals.

1 pound **celeriac** (celery root), peeled and cut into 1-inch cubes

1 pound **rutabaga**, peeled and cut into 1-inch cubes

1 pound **turnips**, peeled and cut into 1-inch cubes

1 large **leek** (white part only), cut in half lengthwise and thinly sliced

4 large cloves **garlic**, thinly sliced

1 cup plain nondairy milk

2 tablespoons vegan butter, or 2 tablespoons **olive oil**

Sea salt

Freshly ground **black** or **white pepper**

Put the celeriac, rutabaga, turnips, leek, and garlic in a large soup pot and cover with water. Cook over medium-high heat until the vegetables are tender, 20 to 25 minutes. Reserve 1½ cups of the cooking liquid. Drain the vegetables in a colander.

Transfer the vegetables to a food processor. Add the milk and butter and process for 1 minute. Scrape down the work bowl. Continue to process, adding a little of the reserved cooking liquid as needed, until the mixture forms a smooth and creamy purée. Season with salt and pepper to taste. Serve hot.

MAKES 6 SERVINGS

Per serving:

133 calories

4 g protein

5 g fat (1 g sat)

20 g carbs

171 mg sodium

145 mg calcium

5 g fiber

Note: Analysis doesn't include sea salt or freshly ground black pepper.

mediterranean roasted vegetables
WITH HERB-ALMOND AIOLI

MAKES 4 SERVINGS

Per serving:

338 calories

2 g protein

25 g fat (3 g sat)

29 g carbs

391 mg sodium

142 mg calcium

8 g fiber

This Mediterranean-inspired dish is made with eggplant, bell peppers, red onion, zucchini, and artichoke hearts, which are all coated with olive oil and seasonings and then oven roasted until fragrant and tender. While this colorful blend of vegetables tastes delicious on its own, the flavor is further enhanced with a topping of Herb-Almond Aioli.

1 **eggplant** (1 to 1¼ pounds), cut into 1-inch cubes

1 **orange or yellow bell pepper**, cut into 1-inch pieces

1 **red bell pepper**, cut into 1-inch pieces

1 large red **onion**, cut into ¼-inch-thick half-moons

1 large **zucchini** or **yellow squash**, cut in half lengthwise and sliced into ½-inch-thick half-moons

2 tablespoons minced **garlic**

2 tablespoons **olive oil**

1½ teaspoons dried rosemary

1 teaspoon dried **basil**

1 teaspoon dried **oregano** or marjoram

Sea salt

Freshly ground **black pepper**

1 can (14 ounces) **artichoke hearts**, cut in half, or 1½ cups frozen artichoke heart pieces, thawed

⅓ cup chopped fresh **parsley**, lightly packed

1 cup Herb-Almond Aioli (page 52)

Preheat the oven to 400 degrees F. Line a baking sheet with parchment paper or a silicone baking mat.

Put the eggplant, orange bell pepper, red bell pepper, onion, zucchini, garlic, oil, rosemary, basil, and oregano in a large bowl and stir until the vegetables are evenly coated. Transfer to the lined baking sheet and spread into a single layer. Sprinkle with salt and pepper as desired. Bake for 25 minutes.

Note: Analysis doesn't include sea salt or freshly ground black pepper.

Remove from the oven. Stir, then spread into a single layer again. Scatter the artichoke hearts over the top. Bake for 10 to 15 minutes longer, or until the vegetables are tender and lightly browned around the edges. Sprinkle the parsley over the top. Top each serving with a dollop of the Herb-Almond Aioli. Serve hot.

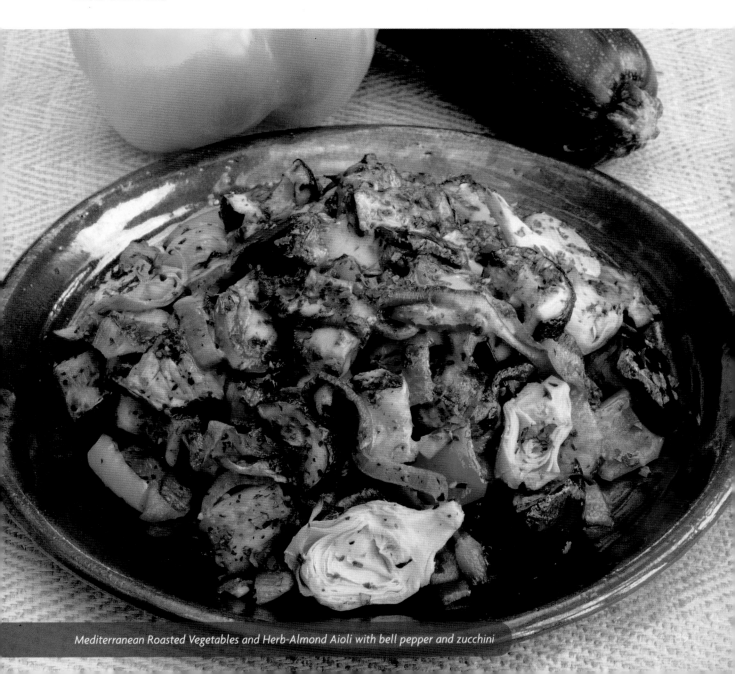

Mediterranean Roasted Vegetables and Herb-Almond Aioli with bell pepper and zucchini

maple-glazed SQUASH

MAKES 6 SERVINGS

Per serving:

106 calories

1 g protein

5 g fat (2 g sat)

22 g carbs

9 mg sodium

43 mg calcium

2 g fiber

Winter squashes abound during the colder months of the year. To make the most of this bounty, give this simple, quick recipe a try. It features tender cubes of winter squash covered in a spiced glaze made with maple syrup and coconut oil.

1 large (about 3 pounds) **winter squash** (such as buttercup, butternut, kabocha, or red kuri), **peeled, seeded, and cut into 1-inch cubes**

1½ **cups water**

1½ **tablespoons peeled and grated fresh ginger**

3 **tablespoons maple syrup**

1 tablespoon **coconut oil**, melted

1 teaspoon ground **cinnamon**

Sea salt

Put the squash, water, and ginger in a large cast-iron or nonstick skillet. Cover and cook over medium heat until the squash is tender, 15 to 20 minutes. Remove the lid. Add the maple syrup, oil, and cinnamon and cook, stirring occasionally, until the cooking liquid thickens to a glaze. Remove from the heat. Season with salt to taste. Serve hot.

> **MAPLE MASHED SQUASH:** Use a potato masher to mash the cooked squash as desired. For an ultracreamy mash, process the mixture in a food processor or use an electric mixer.

Note: Analysis doesn't include sea salt.

SPICY sweet potato fries

Oven-baked fries use just a fraction of the fat as their deep-fried counterparts, which means you can still get your French-fry fix but with less guilt. For a first-rate batch of oven-baked fries, coat sweet potato strips generously with a blend of spices, then bake them until crisp and tender. Chipotle-Almond Mayo (page 52) is an excellent dipping sauce for these spicy fries.

MAKES 4 SERVINGS

Per serving:

200 calories

4 g protein

6 g fat (1 g sat)

35 g carbs

566 mg sodium

56 mg calcium

6 g fiber

5 cups (2 large) **sweet potatoes**, scrubbed well and cut into 3 x ½-inch French fries

1½ tablespoons **olive oil**

1½ tablespoons nutritional yeast flakes

2 teaspoons **chili powder**

1 teaspoon ground **cumin**

1 teaspoon **garlic powder**

¾ teaspoon sea salt

½ teaspoon freshly ground **black pepper**

½ teaspoon **cayenne** or chipotle **chile powder**

Preheat the oven to 425 degrees F. Line a baking sheet with parchment paper or a silicone baking mat.

Put the sweet potatoes, oil, nutritional yeast, chili powder, cumin, garlic powder, salt, pepper, and cayenne in a large bowl and stir until the sweet potatoes are evenly coated. Transfer to the lined baking sheet and spread into a single layer. Bake for 20 minutes.

Remove from the oven. Stir, then spread out the sweet potatoes to form a single layer again. Bake for 15 to 20 minutes longer, or until crisp and lightly browned around the edges. Serve hot.

> **CURRIED SWEET POTATO FRIES:** Replace the chili powder and cayenne with 1½ tablespoons curry powder.

ROASTED brussels sprouts

MAKES 4 SERVINGS

Per serving:

84 calories

5 g protein

4 g fat (1 g sat)

10 g carbs

148 mg sodium

43 mg calcium

3 g fiber

Halved Brussels sprouts are tossed with toasted sesame oil, balsamic vinegar, tamari, and seasonings and then oven-roasted until the edges turn golden brown and crispy. Their smoky, salty, tangy flavor will turn Brussels sprouts haters into lovers!

1 pound **Brussels sprouts**

1 tablespoon balsamic vinegar

1 tablespoon reduced-sodium tamari

1 tablespoon toasted sesame oil

1 tablespoon nutritional yeast flakes

1 teaspoon **garlic powder**

1 teaspoon dried thyme

½ teaspoon crushed **red pepper** flakes (optional)

Sea salt

Freshly ground **black pepper**

Preheat the oven to 400 degrees F. Line a baking sheet with parchment paper or a silicone baking mat.

Trim the ends of the Brussels sprouts, remove any tough or yellow outer leaves, and cut each one in half lengthwise. Put the Brussels sprouts, vinegar, tamari, oil, nutritional yeast, garlic powder, thyme, and optional red pepper flakes in a large bowl and stir until the Brussels sprouts are evenly coated.

Transfer to the lined baking sheet and spread into a single layer. Bake for 20 to 25 minutes, until the Brussels sprouts are crisp and golden brown around the edges. Serve hot.

Note: Analysis doesn't include sea salt or freshly ground black pepper.

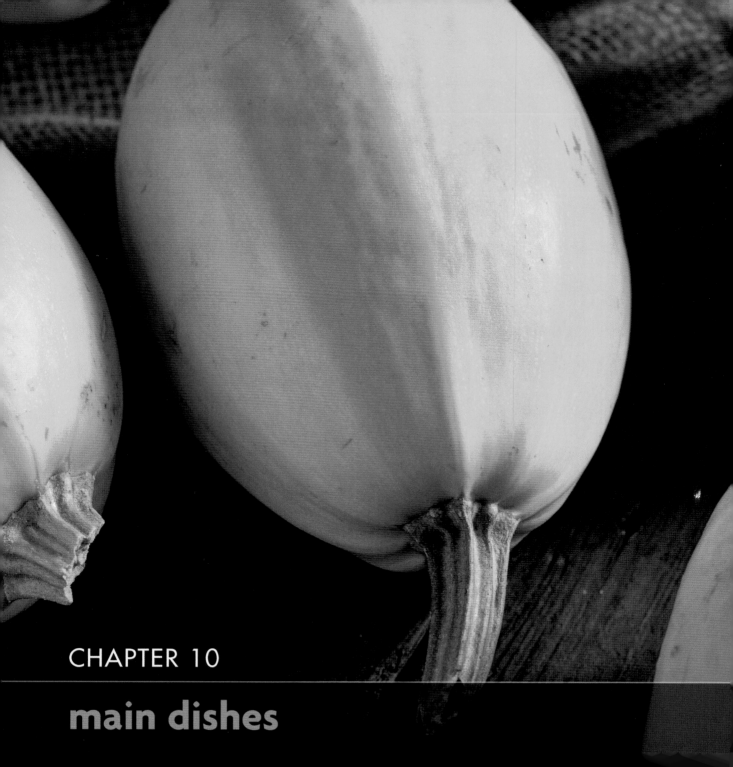

main dishes

walnut-meat SOFT TACOS

MAKES 4 SERVINGS

Per serving:

363 calories

13 g protein

30 g fat (4 g sat)

17 g carbs

302 mg sodium

55 mg calcium

7 g fiber

You'll be amazed by how much the crumbly texture and savory flavor of the walnut taco meat resembles cooked hamburger in this meat-free take on tacos. And if you're gluten-free, you'll be thrilled that lettuce leaves, rather than tortillas, are used to hold the fixin's.

WALNUT TACO MEAT

1 cup raw **walnuts**

1 tablespoon nutritional yeast flakes

1 tablespoon reduced-sodium tamari

1 teaspoon **chili powder**

½ teaspoon ground **cumin**

¼ teaspoon chipotle **chile powder** or **cayenne**

FIXIN'S

1 Hass **avocado**

1 Roma **tomato**, finely diced

6 tablespoons Smoky Cashew Cheese Dip (page 50)

4 large Boston or Bibb lettuce leaves or other lettuce leaves

To make the walnut taco meat, put the walnuts, nutritional yeast, tamari, chili powder, cumin, and chipotle chile powder in a food processor and pulse until the mixture resembles coarse bread crumbs.

For the fixin's, put the avocado in a small bowl and mash with a fork until smooth. Stir in the tomato.

To assemble each taco, put a lettuce leaf on a cutting board, rib-side up. Put ¼ cup of the walnut taco meat in the center of the leaf. Top with 1½ tablespoons of the Smoky Cashew Cheese Dip and one-quarter of the avocado mixture. Repeat the process with the remaining lettuce leaves, walnut taco meat, and fixin's. Serve immediately.

tempeh reuben COLLARD ROLLS

Savory strips of tempeh, cooked sauerkraut, pickles, and homemade chipotle mayo are layered inside large leaves of collard greens instead of bread to create these meat-free, gluten-free reubens.

MAKES 4 SERVINGS

Per serving:

230 calories

10 g protein

17 g fat (2 g sat)

10 g carbs

841 mg sodium

172 mg calcium

2 g fiber

1 package (8 ounces) **tempeh**

1 tablespoon reduced-sodium tamari

1⅓ cups **Sauerkraut** (page 48), drained

2 tablespoons **olive oil**

6 tablespoons Chipotle-Almond Mayo (page 52)

4 slices Refrigerator Garlic-Dill Sandwich Pickles (page 49)

4 large leaves **collard greens**, bottom stems trimmed flush with the leaves

Cut the tempeh into quarters lengthwise, then slice each piece horizontally to yield a total of 8 pieces. Transfer to a baking dish. Pour the tamari over the tempeh and let marinate for 10 minutes.

Put the sauerkraut and ½ tablespoon of the oil in a large cast-iron or nonstick skillet and cook over medium-high heat, stirring occasionally, until the sauerkraut is dry and lightly browned, 2 to 3 minutes. Transfer to a large plate.

Put the tempeh and remaining 1½ tablespoons of oil in the same skillet. Cook over medium-high heat until lightly browned, about 5 minutes. Flip over the tempeh and cook until lightly browned on the other side, 3 to 5 minutes.

To assemble each roll, put 1 collard leaf, rib-side up, on a cutting board. Spread 1½ tablespoons of the Chipotle-Almond Mayo in the center of the leaf. On top of the mayo put 2 tempeh pieces, ⅓ cup of the sauerkraut, and 1 pickle slice. Fold the stem end and top edge of the collard leaf toward the center. Fold in the right side tightly over the filling, then fold in and overlap the left side of the leaf. Repeat the process with the remaining collard leaves and fillings. Serve immediately.

spaghetti squash
WITH ROASTED RED PEPPER SAUCE

MAKES 4 SERVINGS

Per serving:

138 calories

4 g protein

8 fat (1 g sat)

17 g carbs

32 mg sodium

56 mg calcium

3 g fiber

Spaghetti squash is aptly named because raking the inside with a fork quickly transforms it into long, spaghetti-like strands. For this mock-pasta recipe, cooked strands of spaghetti squash are topped with a sweet-and-spicy roasted red pepper sauce and fresh basil. It's sure to please!

1 large **spaghetti squash**, cut in half lengthwise and seeded

2 large red **bell peppers**, cut into 2-inch pieces

2 **shallots**, chopped, or 1 yellow **onion**, cut into 2-inch pieces

5 whole cloves **garlic**, peeled

2 tablespoons **olive oil**

⅔ cup low-sodium vegetable broth

2 tablespoons nutritional yeast flakes

¾ teaspoon sweet or smoked **paprika**

Sea salt

Freshly ground **black pepper**

3 tablespoons chopped fresh **basil** or **parsley**

Crushed **red pepper** flakes (optional)

Preheat the oven to 375 degrees F. Line two baking sheets with parchment paper or silicone baking mats.

Put the spaghetti squash, cut-side down, on one of the lined baking sheets. Put the bell peppers, shallots, garlic cloves, and 1 tablespoon of the oil in a large bowl and stir to combine. Transfer the bell peppers to the remaining lined baking sheet and spread into a single layer. Bake the spaghetti squash and bell peppers for 30 minutes.

Remove the baking sheets from the oven. Flip the spaghetti squash over and let the squash and bell peppers cool for 5 minutes.

To make the roasted red pepper sauce, transfer the bell pepper mixture to a blender. Add the remaining tablespoon of oil and the broth, nutritional yeast, and paprika and process until smooth. Season with salt and pepper to taste. Scrape down the blender jar and process for 15 seconds longer.

Note: Analysis doesn't include sea salt or freshly ground black pepper.

Using a fork, rake the cut surface of the squash to separate it into long strands that resemble spaghetti. Transfer the squash strands to a large platter or bowl. Top with the roasted red pepper sauce. Scatter the basil over the sauce. Garnish each serving with red pepper flakes if desired.

black bean and pumpkin CURRY

Large cubes of pumpkin are cooked in vegetable broth, coconut milk, and curry paste to create the luscious base for this sweet-and-spicy curry. The last-minute addition of black beans, red bell pepper, and cilantro contributes a delightful contrast of color and flavor. Serve the curry on its own or over your favorite cooked grain.

1 yellow **onion**, diced

1 tablespoon **coconut oil** or other oil

1 tablespoon red or green **curry paste**

1 small (3 to 4 pounds) **pumpkin**, peeled, seeded, and cut into 1½-inch cubes

1½ cups low-sodium vegetable broth

1 can (14 ounces) lite **coconut milk**

1 can (15 ounces) black beans, drained and rinsed

1 red **bell pepper**, diced

⅓ cup chopped fresh **cilantro** or Thai **basil**, lightly packed

Juice of 1 **lime**

Sea salt

Freshly ground **black pepper**

MAKES 6 SERVINGS

Per serving:

146 calories

5 g protein

7 g fat (6 g sat)

22 g carbs

354 mg sodium

49 mg calcium

5 g fiber

Put the onion and oil in a large soup pot and cook over medium heat, stirring occasionally, for 5 minutes. Add the curry paste and cook, stirring occasionally, for 1 minute.

Add the pumpkin, broth, and coconut milk and stir to combine. Bring to a boil over high heat. Cover, decrease the heat to low, and simmer for 15 minutes.

Add the beans and bell pepper and simmer, stirring occasionally, until the vegetables are tender, 8 to 10 minutes. Remove from the heat. Stir in the cilantro and lime juice. Season with salt and pepper to taste. Serve hot.

Note: Analysis doesn't include sea salt or freshly ground black pepper.

CURRIED tofu and vegetable kabobs

MAKES 4 SERVINGS

Per serving:

353 calories

24 g protein

18 g fat (3 g sat)

28 g carbs

253 mg sodium

180 mg calcium

3 g fiber

These savory kabobs are made with alternating pieces of tofu, broccoli, mushrooms, zucchini, red onion, and bell pepper that have been infused with a curry-flavored marinade. The assembled kabobs can be cooked on either an outdoor grill or grill pan on the stove top.

1 pound extra-firm **tofu**

16 button **mushrooms**

1 **orange or yellow bell pepper**, cut into 16 (1-inch) pieces

16 large **broccoli** florets

1 large **zucchini**, cut into 16 slices

1 **red bell pepper**, cut into 16 (1-inch) pieces

2 red or yellow **onions**, each cut into 8 wedges

⅓ cup low-sodium vegetable broth or water

2 tablespoons **olive oil** or other oil

2 tablespoons agave nectar or maple syrup

Zest and juice of 1 **lime**

1½ tablespoons reduced-sodium tamari

1 tablespoon **curry powder**

1 tablespoon minced **garlic**

1 tablespoon peeled and grated fresh **ginger**

1 teaspoon **hot sauce**

¼ teaspoon freshly ground **black pepper**

Have ready eight bamboo, wooden, or metal skewers. If using bamboo or wooden skewers, soak them in water for at least 30 minutes.

Gently squeeze the block of tofu over the sink to remove any excess water. Cut the tofu into sixteen cubes.

Thread each skewer in this order: one mushroom, one piece orange bell pepper, one broccoli floret, one tofu cube, one slice zucchini, one piece red bell pepper, one wedge onion. Repeat the procedure reversing the order and ending with a mushroom. Arrange the skewers in a single layer in a large baking pan.

To make the marinade, put the broth, oil, agave nectar, lime zest and juice, tamari, curry powder, garlic, ginger, hot sauce, and pepper in a small bowl and whisk to combine. Pour the marinade over the kabobs, rotating them as needed to evenly coat all sides. Cover the baking pan, put it in the refrigerator, and let the tofu and vegetables marinate for 1 hour or longer.

Cook the skewers on a hot oiled grill or grill pan until the tofu and vegetables are lightly charred all over, 2 to 3 minutes per side. Serve hot.

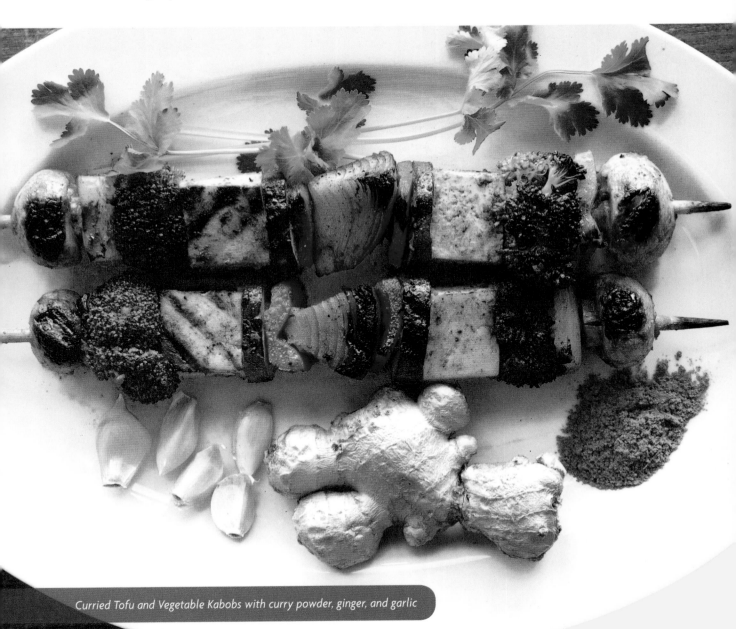

Curried Tofu and Vegetable Kabobs with curry powder, ginger, and garlic

nut-crusted tofu cutlets WITH CASHEW GRAVY

MAKES 4 SERVINGS

Per serving:

534 calories

33 g protein

35 g fat (6 g sat)

32 g carbs

672 mg sodium

265 mg calcium

12 g fiber

Finely grinding nuts with seasonings in a food processor transforms them into a mixture resembling bread crumbs. In this recipe they're used to coat marinated tofu, which is then oven baked until golden brown and crispy. To amplify the nutty flavor even more, the tofu is topped with a savory cashew gravy.

1 pound extra-firm **tofu**

3 tablespoons plain nondairy milk

1 tablespoon reduced-sodium tamari

1 teaspoon cider vinegar

1 cup raw nuts (such as **almonds**, hazelnuts, or pecans)

2 tablespoons nutritional yeast flakes

1 teaspoon **garlic powder**

1 teaspoon **onion powder**

½ teaspoon sweet or smoked **paprika**

½ teaspoon sea salt

¼ teaspoon freshly ground **black pepper**

2½ cups Savory Cashew Gravy (page 51)

Gently squeeze the block of tofu over the sink to remove any excess water. Cut the tofu lengthwise into eight slices and arrange them in a single layer in an 11 x 7-inch baking pan. Using a fork, pierce each tofu slice several times along its length. Flip each slice over and pierce the other side.

To make the marinade, put the milk, tamari, and vinegar in a small bowl and stir to combine. Pour the mixture over the tofu and flip each slice to evenly coat all sides. Put the baking pan in the refrigerator and let the tofu marinate for 1 hour or longer.

To make the nut crumbs, put the nuts, nutritional yeast, garlic powder, onion powder, paprika, salt, and pepper in a food processor and process until the nuts are finely ground. Transfer to a large plate.

Preheat the oven to 400 degrees F. Line a baking sheet with parchment paper or a silicone baking mat.

To coat the tofu, work with one slice at a time. Put each slice into the nut mixture, pressing it down lightly and flipping it over as needed until all sides are evenly coated. Transfer to the lined baking sheet.

Bake for 20 minutes. Remove from the oven and flip the cutlets over. Bake for 15 to 20 minutes longer, until golden brown. Top with the cashew gravy or pass the gravy at the table. Serve hot.

mac-n-cheese cauliflower CASSEROLE

Steamed cauliflower by itself is somewhat bland and boring. But when it's bathed in a cashew-based cheese sauce, it's transformed into a mouthwatering pasta-free mac-n-cheese casserole that young and old alike will love.

1 large head (2½ to 3 pounds) **cauliflower**, cut into florets

⅔ cup water

Sea salt

Freshly ground **black pepper**

3 cups Cashew Cheese Sauce or Spicy Nacho Cheese Sauce (page 50)

⅔ cup coarsely chopped raw **walnuts**

2 tablespoons chopped fresh **parsley**

Sweet or smoked **paprika**

MAKES 4 SERVINGS

Per serving:

798 calories

43 g protein

49 g fat (7 g sat)

56 g carbs

992 mg sodium

110 mg calcium

19 g fiber

Preheat the oven to 375 degrees F. Lightly oil an 11 x 7-inch baking pan or mist it with cooking spray.

Put the cauliflower and water in a large pot. Cover and cook over medium-high heat until the cauliflower is tender, 8 to 10 minutes. Drain and transfer to a large bowl. Season with salt and pepper to taste.

Add the Cashew Cheese Sauce and stir until evenly distributed. Transfer the mixture to the prepared baking pan. Bake for 20 minutes.

Remove from the oven. Scatter the walnuts and parsley over the cauliflower mixture. Sprinkle a little paprika over the top. Bake for 10 to 15 minutes longer, until the walnuts are fragrant and golden brown.

> **VARIATION:** Replace the fresh cauliflower with 2 packages (16 ounces each) frozen cauliflower florets, thawed.

Note: Analysis doesn't include sea salt or freshly ground black pepper.

broccoli rabe and white beans
WITH ZUCCHINI NOODLES

MAKES 4 SERVINGS

Per serving:

213 calories

15 g protein

6 g fat (1 g sat)

27 g carbs

305 mg sodium

238 mg calcium

9 g fiber

Broccoli rabe, also known as rapini, is a cruciferous vegetable with edible stems, leaves, and small broccoli-like florets that are slightly bitter. For this Italian-inspired dish, broccoli rabe is quickly cooked in olive oil, along with white beans and a generous amount of garlic, before being tossed with zucchini noodles.

2 large **zucchini** or **yellow squashes**

1 bunch (about 1½ pounds) **broccoli rabe**, cut into 1-inch pieces

1½ tablespoons **olive oil**

1 can (15 ounces) **white beans** (such as cannellini, navy, or white kidney), drained and rinsed

3 tablespoons minced **garlic**

1 teaspoon dried **basil**

1 teaspoon dried **oregano**

½ teaspoon crushed **red pepper** flakes (optional)

1½ tablespoons nutritional yeast flakes

Sea salt

Freshly ground **black pepper**

Use a spiralizer to cut the zucchini into thin or thick spaghetti strands, then cut the strands with a knife into 4-inch lengths. Alternatively, use a vegetable peeler to shave long strips down the entire length of each zucchini. When the center seed section is reached, turn the zucchini and shave strips from another side. Continue in this fashion until all sides are shaved.

Put the broccoli rabe and oil in a large cast-iron or nonstick skillet and cook over medium-high heat, stirring occasionally, for 5 minutes. Add the beans, garlic, basil, oregano, and optional red pepper flakes and cook, stirring occasionally, until the broccoli rabe is crisp-tender, 2 to 3 minutes. Add the zucchini noodles and nutritional yeast and toss until evenly distributed. Season with salt and pepper to taste. Serve hot.

Note: Analysis doesn't include sea salt or freshly ground black pepper.

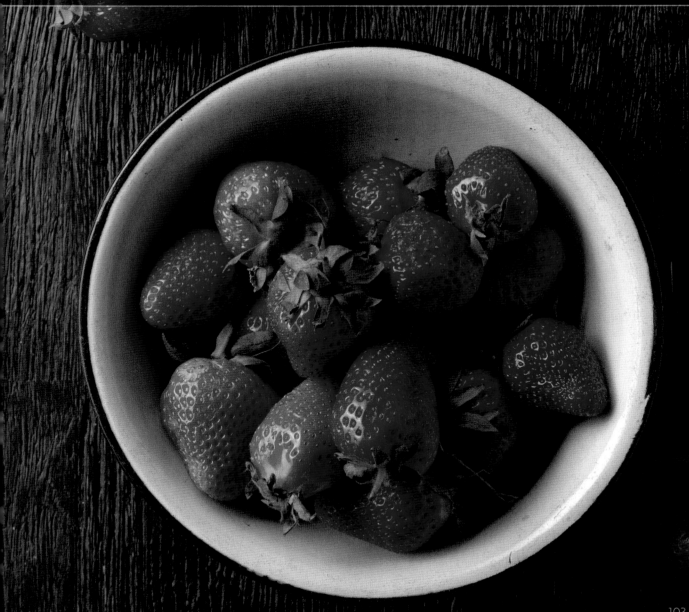

sweet treats

minty melon SORBET

MAKES 4 SERVINGS

Per serving:

85 calories

1 g protein

0 g fat (0 g sat)

21 g carbs

39 mg sodium

31 mg calcium

2 g fiber

Sorbet is a light and refreshing dessert as well as a guilt-free indulgence after a heavy, rich, or spicy meal. It's also a welcome treat during the sweltering summer months. This sorbet is made without any added sweetener, so it tastes best when made with fully ripe or overripe melon.

4 cups melon (such as cantaloupe, crenshaw, honeydew, or watermelon), **cut into 1-inch cubes**

½ cup **apple juice** or white **grape juice**

¼ cup chopped fresh **mint**, lightly packed

2 tablespoons **lime or lemon juice**

Put all the ingredients in a food processor or blender and process until smooth. Scrape down the work bowl or blender jar and process for 15 seconds longer. Spoon into an airtight container, cover, and freeze for 30 minutes.

Return the mixture to the food processor or blender and process for 30 seconds to break up any ice crystals. Transfer the mixture back to the container. Cover and freeze until firm, 3 to 4 hours.

> **VARIATION:** Replace the melon with 4 cups cubed fresh fruit (such as mangoes, nectarines, oranges, peaches, or pineapple), berries, or pitted cherries.

cherry-almond chia pudding WITH DRIED FRUIT

Cherries and almonds are members of the rose family, and their flavors go together like best friends. Chia seeds are the secret ingredient in this uncooked pudding, as they create a thick, creamy consistency. Each serving is topped with sweet, chewy dried figs and mulberries.

1½ cups pitted sweet or sour **cherries**, cut in half, or 1 package (10 ounces) frozen cherries, thawed, drained, and cut in half

⅔ cup coarsely chopped raw **almonds**

¼ cup coarsely chopped dried figs

¼ cup dried **mulberries**

2 cups water

4 pitted soft dates

1 tablespoon peeled and grated fresh **ginger**

1 tablespoon vanilla extract

3 tablespoons **chia seeds**

MAKES 4 SERVINGS

Per serving:

296 calories

7 g protein

12 g fat (1 g sat)

42 g carbs

15 mg sodium

124 mg calcium

7 g fiber

Put ¼ cup of the cherries and 2 tablespoons of the almonds in a small bowl. Add the figs and mulberries and stir to combine. Set aside.

Put the remaining cherries and almonds in a blender. Add the water, dates, ginger, and vanilla extract and process until smooth, about 1 minute. Scrape down the blender jar. Add the chia seeds and process until well combined, about 15 seconds.

Transfer to a medium glass or ceramic bowl and refrigerate until the chia seeds swell and thicken the mixture into a pudding, about 1 hour.

Before serving, whisk the mixture to break up any clumps of chia seeds. Top each serving with one-quarter of the reserved fruit mixture. Serve immediately.

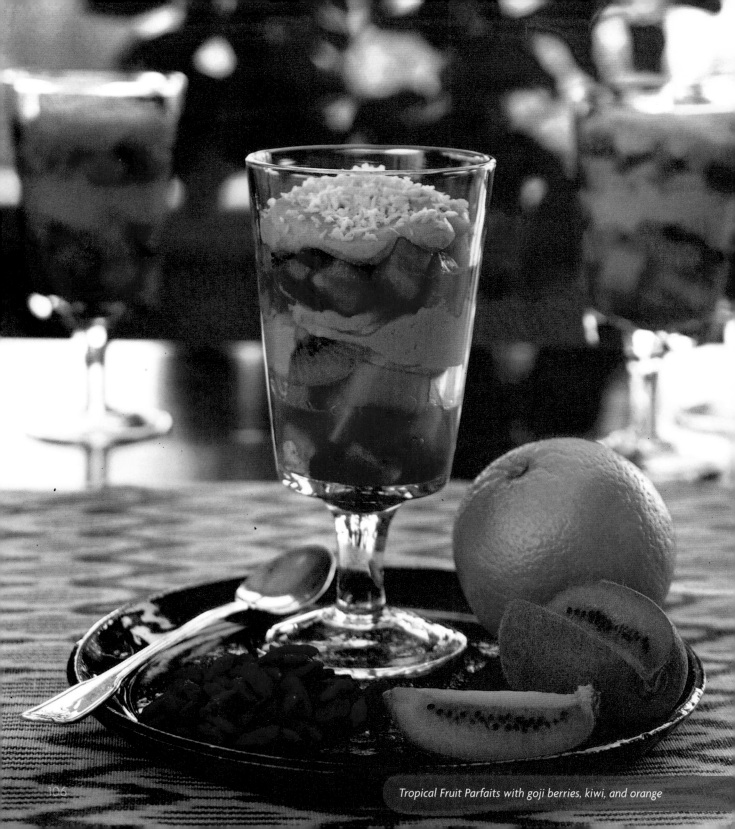

Tropical Fruit Parfaits with goji berries, kiwi, and orange

TROPICAL fruit parfaits

One bite of these gorgeous parfaits and your taste buds will travel to a tropical island paradise without ever leaving home. They're made with alternating layers of vanilla-infused, nut-based whipped topping and a luscious blend of goji berries, kiwi, mango, and papaya, all of which are anti-inflammatory superstars.

Juice of 1 **orange**

⅓ cup **goji berries**

1 **papaya**, peeled and diced

1 **mango**, peeled and diced

2 **kiwi**, peeled, quartered lengthwise, and thinly sliced

1½ cups Vanilla-Nut Whipped Topping (page 114)

2 tablespoons unsweetened shredded dried **coconut**

MAKES 4 SERVINGS

Per serving:

683 calories

10 g protein

42 g fat (8 g sat)

86 g carbs

25 mg sodium

108 mg calcium

14 g fiber

Put the orange juice and goji berries in medium bowl and set aside for 5 minutes to rehydrate the goji berries. Add the papaya, mango, and kiwi, and stir to combine.

Have ready four large glasses or dessert dishes. To assemble each parfait, layer one-eighth of the fruit mixture and 3 tablespoons of the Vanilla-Nut Whipped Topping in the bottom of each glass or dessert dish. Repeat the layers, then top with ½ tablespoon of the shredded coconut. Serve immediately.

VARIATION: Replace any of the suggested fruits with other tropical fruits, such as dragon fruit, guava, passion fruit, or star fruit.

trail mix COOKIES

MAKES 20 COOKIES

Per cookie:

145 calories

3 g protein

7 g fat (1 g sat)

18 g carbs

48 mg sodium

23 mg calcium

3 g fiber

Rather than rolled oats, these cookies are made with a combination of pulverized steel-cut oats and intact pieces, which enhances their texture. These tasty cookies are accented with dried fruit, shredded coconut, and pumpkin and sunflower seeds. Although specific amounts of each are suggested, they all can be replaced with one cup of your favorite trail mix.

3 tablespoons warm water

1 teaspoon **chia seeds**, or 1 tablespoon ground **flaxseeds** or **flaxseed meal**

2½ cups steel-cut oats

¾ teaspoon ground **cinnamon**

½ teaspoon ground **ginger**

½ teaspoon baking soda

¼ teaspoon sea salt

¼ cup maple syrup or agave nectar

¼ cup sunflower seed butter or tahini

¼ cup sunflower oil or canola oil

1 teaspoon vanilla extract

½ cup mixed dried fruit (such as **cherries**, **cranberries**, **goji berries**, **mulberries**, or raisins)

¼ cup unsweetened shredded dried **coconut**

3 tablespoons raw **pumpkin seeds**

2 tablespoons raw sunflower seeds

Preheat the oven to 350 degrees F. Line two baking sheets with parchment paper or silicone baking mats.

Put the water and chia seeds in a small bowl and whisk vigorously to combine. Let rest for 10 minutes until the mixture thickens into a gel.

Put 2 cups of the steel-cut oats in a blender and process into a fine flour, about 1 minute. Transfer the oat flour to a large bowl. Add the remaining ½ cup of steel-cut oats and the cinnamon, ginger, baking soda, and salt and stir to combine.

Add the chia seed gel, maple syrup, sunflower seed butter, oil, and vanilla extract and stir to combine. Gently stir in the dried fruit, coconut, pumpkin seeds, and sunflower seeds.

Portion the dough onto the lined baking sheets using a 1½-inch ice-cream scoop or 1 heaping tablespoon per cookie, spacing them 2 inches apart. Slightly flatten each cookie with wet fingers.

Bake for 8 to 10 minutes, until the tops feel dry. Let cool completely on the baking sheets.

seared pineapple WITH DATE CARAMEL SAUCE

Searing slices of fresh pineapple in a dry skillet until golden brown caramelizes the natural sugars and enhances the sweetness of this succulent fruit. While seared pineapple tastes delish on its own, it's even better when topped with a sumptuous date-based sauce. Although the sauce is sugar-free, it tastes surprisingly like caramel.

1¼ cups **coconut water**

½ cup pitted soft dates

1 tablespoon **coconut oil**

1 tablespoon vanilla extract

1 **pineapple**, peeled, cored, and cut into 8 slices

MAKES 4 SERVINGS

Per serving:

171 calories

2 g protein

4 g fat (3 g sat)

40 g carbs

18 mg sodium

50 mg calcium

1 g fiber

To make the sauce, put the coconut water, dates, oil, and vanilla extract in a blender and process until smooth, 1 to 2 minutes. Scrape down the blender jar and process for 15 seconds longer.

Put a large cast-iron or nonstick skillet over medium-high heat. Put four pineapple slices in the hot skillet and cook until the bottoms are golden brown, 2 to 3 minutes. Flip the slices over and cook until golden brown on the other side, 1 to 2 minutes. Transfer to a large plate. Repeat the process with the remaining pineapple slices.

For each serving, put two pineapple-slices on a plate and top with ⅓ cup of the date caramel sauce. Serve immediately.

STEWED rhubarb and strawberries

To help counterbalance the tartness of rhubarb, it's paired with sweet, juicy strawberries along with cardamom, ginger, and lemon. Agave nectar is added to taste, as the tartness of rhubarb and strawberries can vary greatly depending on how ripe they are. Enjoy this as a dessert, breakfast, or side dish, plain or topped with nondairy ice cream or yogurt. Alternatively, use it to top cake, pancakes, toast, or waffles.

> 1 pound (6 to 8 large stalks) fresh **rhubarb**, cut into 1-inch pieces
>   (about 4 cups)
>
> Zest and juice of 1 **lemon**
>
> 1½ tablespoons peeled and grated fresh **ginger**
>
> 1 teaspoon ground **cardamom** or **cinnamon**
>
> 1 pint **strawberries**, hulled and cut in half
>
> ⅓ cup agave nectar, plus more as needed

Put the rhubarb, lemon zest and juice, ginger, and cardamom in a medium saucepan and stir to combine. Bring to a boil over high heat. Decrease the heat to low and simmer for 15 minutes.

Add the strawberries and agave nectar and cook, stirring occasionally, until the fruit is soft, 10 to 15 minutes. Taste and add additional agave nectar as desired. Serve hot, warm, or cold.

> **TIP:** Only the celery-like stalks of rhubarb are edible. Never eat the leafy tops, as they can be toxic. For the sweetest rhubarb, choose deep-red stalks.

> **VARIATION:** If fresh rhubarb and strawberries aren't available, replace them with 1 pound frozen sliced rhubarb and 1 pound frozen whole strawberries.

raw stone fruit CRUMBLE

During the hot summer months, the last thing most cooks want to do is heat up the oven to make a dessert. This no-bake fruit crumble is ideal for those times. Using very ripe fruit is a must for this dessert. Serve it plain or topped with Vanilla-Nut Whipped Topping (page 114) or nondairy ice cream.

½ cup **coconut water** or water

6 pitted soft dates

1 cup raw **walnuts** or other nuts

⅓ cup unsweetened shredded dried **coconut**

1 teaspoon ground **cinnamon**

¼ teaspoon freshly grated nutmeg

4 **nectarines** or **peaches**, or 3 cups sliced **apricots**, **plums**, or **pluots**

1 teaspoon vanilla extract

½ teaspoon ground **ginger** or **cardamom**

MAKES 4 SERVINGS

Per serving:

411 calories

7 g protein

23 g fat (6 g sat)

50 g carbs

10 mg sodium

62 mg calcium

6 g fiber

Put the coconut water and dates in a small bowl. Set aside for 10 minutes to rehydrate the dates.

To make the crumble mixture, put four of the dates and the walnuts, coconut, cinnamon, and nutmeg in a food processor. Pulse until the mixture resembles coarse bread crumbs. Transfer to a small bowl and set aside.

To make the sauce, dice one of nectarines and put it in the food processor. If using sliced fruit, use 1 cup for the sauce. Add the vanilla extract, ginger, and the remaining two dates (save the soaking liquid) and process into a slightly chunky purée. Scrape down the work bowl. Continue processing, adding some of the soaking liquid as needed, until the mixture is smooth and saucy.

To assemble the crumble, slice the remaining 3 nectarines and put them in a 9-inch baking pan. Pour the sauce over the top and stir to evenly coat the fruit. Sprinkle the crumble mixture evenly over the top. Serve immediately or well chilled.

mexican hot chocolate cake
WITH CACAO NIBS AND NUTS

MAKES 9 SERVINGS

Per serving:

391 calories

10 g protein

31 g fat (3 g sat)

28 g carbs

140 mg sodium

105 mg calcium

7 g fiber

Warm and stimulating Mexican hot chocolate, which is typically enhanced with ground cinnamon and chiles, provided the inspiration for this gluten-free cake. Chia gel helps bind the batter of this dark-chocolate confection, which is topped with chopped nuts and cacao nibs. Serve with a scoop of your favorite vegan ice cream on the side.

¼ cup warm water

1½ teaspoons **chia seeds**

3 cups **almond flour**

6 tablespoons **cacao powder** or unsweetened cocoa powder

2 teaspoons baking soda

1 teaspoon ground **cinnamon**

¾ teaspoon **cayenne** or chipotle **chile powder**

½ teaspoon sea salt

½ cup agave nectar or maple syrup

6 tablespoons canola or other oil

1 teaspoon vanilla extract

⅓ cup coarsely chopped nuts (such as **almonds**, Brazil nuts, hazelnuts, pecans, or **walnuts**)

¼ cup cacao nibs

Preheat the oven to 350 degrees F. Lightly oil a 9-inch square baking pan or mist it with cooking spray.

Put the water and chia seeds in a small bowl and whisk vigorously to combine. Let rest for 10 minutes, until the mixture thickens into a gel.

Put the almond flour, cacao powder, baking powder, cinnamon, cayenne, and salt in a large bowl and whisk to combine. Add the chia seed gel, agave nectar, oil, and vanilla extract and whisk to combine. The batter will be very thick.

Transfer the batter to the prepared baking pan. Scatter the chopped nuts and cacao nibs over the top and use a spatula to gently press them into the batter. Bake for 30 to 35 minutes, or until a toothpick inserted in the center comes out clean. Let cool completely before slicing and serving.

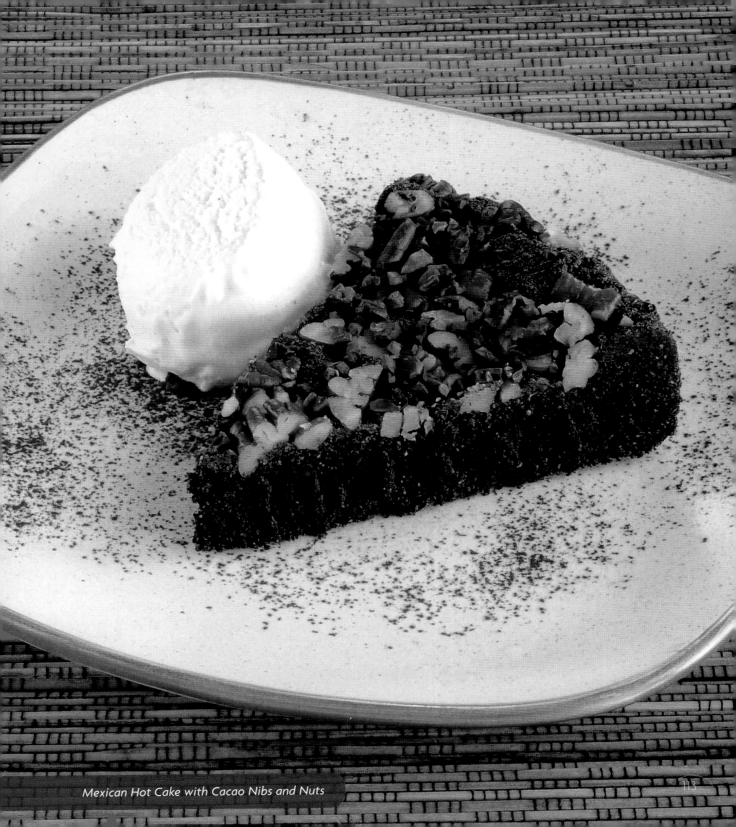

Mexican Hot Cake with Cacao Nibs and Nuts

vanilla-nut WHIPPED TOPPING

MAKES 1½ CUPS

Per 2 tablespoons:

154 calories

2 g protein

13 g fat (2 g sat)

11 g carbs

1 mg sodium

22 mg calcium

2 g fiber

Soaked macadamia nuts and dates are blended with a touch of vanilla extract to create this light and creamy topping. Use it in lieu of whipped cream on sliced fresh fruit or berries or your favorite desserts.

> 2½ cups warm water
>
> 1½ cups raw **macadamia nuts**
>
> 6 pitted soft dates
>
> 1½ teaspoons vanilla extract

Put 2 cups of the water and the macadamia nuts in a medium bowl. Put the dates and remaining ½ cup of water in a small bowl. Let the nuts and dates soak for 1 hour or longer. Drain the macadamia nuts but do not drain the dates.

Put the macadamia nuts, the dates and their soaking liquid, and the vanilla extract in a blender and process until smooth. Scrape down the blender jar and process until thick and creamy, 3 to 5 minutes. Stored in an airtight container in the refrigerator, the topping will keep for 5 days. Serve cold.

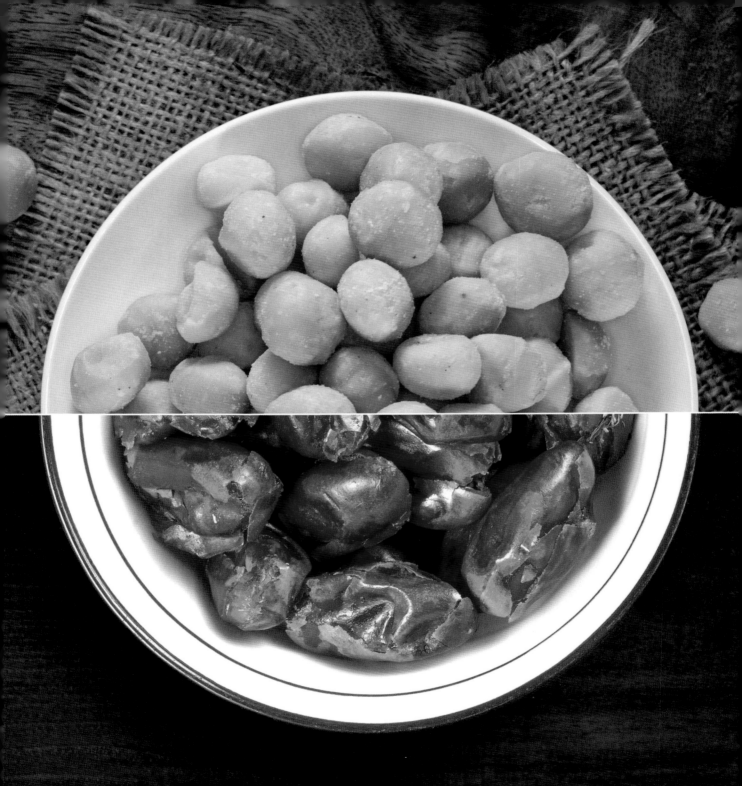

Recipe titles appear in *italics*.

A

açaí berries, as anti-inflammatory, 26
active fighters, 4–5
acute inflammation, 1, 2, 7, 8
advanced glycation end products (AGES), 11
AGES (advanced glycation end products), 11
aging, 9–10, 12
Aioli, Herb-Almond, Mediterranean Roasted Vegetables with, 88–89
alcohol consumption, avoiding, 20–21
alkaloids, 20, 28
allergies
  antihistamines and, 17
  autoimmune diseases and, 9
  histamine and, 3
  as inflammatory response, 2
  latex and, 27
  nuts and, 26
  tropical fruits and, 27
allium vegetables, as anti-inflammatory, 28
almond(s)
  aioli, herb-almond, 52
    Mediterranean Roasted Vegetables with, 88–89
  as anti-inflammatory, 25
  Chia Pudding, Cherry-Almond, with Dried Fruit, 105
  Green and Yellow Beans Amandine, 83
  Mayo, Chipotle-Almond, 52
  milk tea, almond (or coconut), 34
Alzheimer's disease, 8, 18, 22, 23, 31
anaphylaxis, 2
Ancient Grains, Mushroom, and Asparagus Medley, 75
anthocyanins, 20, 26
antihistamines, 17

The Anti-Inflammation Zone (Sears), 5
anti-inflammatory foods
  chocolate, 30
  fruits, 26–28
  green tea, 30
  herbs/spices, 30–32
  seeds, nuts, and oils, 25–26
  using in recipes, 32
  vegetables, 28–30
anti-inflammatory prostaglandins, 20
anti-inflammatory reaction, 2, 3, 10, 22
antioxidants, 5, 23, 27, 29, 30
apples, as anti-inflammatory, 27
arachidonic acid, 8, 11, 15, 21
arthritis
  cashews and, 26
  chronic inflammation and, 8
  nightshade fruits/vegetables and, 20, 28
  pineapple and, 27
  piperine and, 31
  steroids and, 18
Asparagus, Ancient Grains, and Mushroom Medley, 75
asthma, 9, 26
autoimmune diseases, 8–9
avocados, as anti-inflammatory, 27–28

B

basil, as anti-inflammatory, 31
Bavarian Slaw, 54
beans, protein in, 21–23. *See also* specific types of beans
beet(s) (or beet greens)
  as anti-inflammatory, 29
  Borscht, 65
  Gold Beet "Rice," Mexican-Style, 76
  in hash recipe, 46
  in slaw recipe, 55

bell peppers, inflammation and, 28
berry(ies). *See also* specific types of
  as anti-inflammatory, 26–27
  Berrylicious Spinach Salad, with Raspberry Chia-Poppy Seed Dressing, 58
  Smoothie, Blast-Off, 35
beta-carotene, 28, 29
beverages
  Berry Blast-Off Smoothie, 35
  Go Green Tea Smoothie, 37
  Golden Milk Tea, 34
  Nutty Chocolate Smoothie, 36
Black Bean and Pumpkin Curry, 97
Black Beans, Mayan, 81
black pepper, as anti-inflammatory, 31
Blast-Off Smoothie, Berry, 35
Blender Oat Pancakes, 41
blueberries, as anti-inflammatory, 26
bok choy, as anti-inflammatory, 29
Borscht, 65
Bowl, Superfood Smoothie, 38
breakfast
  Grits, Paleo, 42
  Oat Pancakes, Blender, 41
  Oats Porridge, Steel-Cut, 40
  Red Flannel Hash, 46
  Superfood Smoothie Bowl, 38
  Sweet Potato Breakfast Skillet, Creole-Style, 45
  Tofu Scramble, Indian-Style, 43
breast cancer, foods to fight against, 25, 27
Broccoli and Cauliflower Soup, Creamy, 68
Broccoli Rabe and White Beans with Zucchini Noodles, 102
Brussels sprouts
  as anti-inflammatory, 29
  in *Bavarian Slaw*, 54
  Roasted, 92

C

cabbage
    as anti-inflammatory, 29
    Napa, and Vegetable Salad, Shredded, 56
    Sauerkraut, 48
    Slaw, Bavarian, 54
Cacao Nibs and Nuts, Mexican Hot Chocolate Cake with, 112
caffeine consumption, avoiding, 20
Cake, Mexican Hot Chocolate, with Cacao Nibs and Nuts, 112
cancer
    açaí berries and, 26
    anti-inflammatory drugs and, 18
    chronic inflammation and, 8
    coding in cells and, 9
    cucumber and, 29
    fish oil and, 18, 22
    fruits and, 27
    garlic and, 28
    herbs/spices and, 31, 32
    mushrooms and, 30
    omega-3 and, 18
    pineapple and, 27
    red meat consumption and, 12
    sauerkraut and, 29
    walnuts and, 25
Caramel Sauce, Date, Seared Pineapple with, 109
cardamom, as anti-inflammatory, 31
carotenoids, 20, 27, 28
carrots, as anti-inflammatory, 29
carrots, in slaw recipes, 54, 55
cashew(s)
    as anti-inflammatory, 25–26
    cheese dip, smoky, 50
    Cheese Sauce, 50
    gravy
        mushroom-, 51
        Nut-Crusted Tofu Cutlets with, 100–101
        Savory, 51
    Pineapple and, Cauliflower Fried "Rice" with, 77
Casserole, Mac-n-Cheese Cauliflower, 101
cauliflower
    as anti-inflammatory, 29
    and Broccoli Soup, Creamy, 68
    Casserole, Mac-n-Cheese, 101
    Fried "Rice" with Pineapple and Cashews, 77
cayenne, inflammation and, 28
celeriac, as anti-inflammatory, 30
celery, as anti-inflammatory, 30
cereal recipes, 40, 42

chard, as anti-inflammatory, 29
cheese
    dip, smoky cashew, 50
    Mac-n-Cheese Cauliflower Casserole, 101
    Sauce, Cashew, 50
    sauce, spicy nacho, 50
cherries, as anti-inflammatory, 26
Cherry Tomato and Squash Medley with Olives, 86
Cherry-Almond Chia Pudding with Dried Fruit, 105
chia seeds
    as anti-inflammatory, 25
    Chia Pudding, Cherry-Almond, with Dried Fruit, 105
    Chia-Poppy Seed Raspberry Dressing, Berrylicious Spinach Salad with, 58
    omega-3s in, 19, 22, 25
chile peppers, inflammation and, 28
chiles and green onions, paleo grits with, 42
Chili, Mexicali Veggie, 70–71
chipotle(s)
    -Almond Mayo, 52
    Pumpkin-Chipotle Soup, Smoky, 69
    tip about, 69
chocolate
    as anti-inflammatory, 30
    Cake, Mexican Hot Chocolate, with Cacao Nibs and Nuts, 112
    Smoothie, Nutty, 36
chronic inflammation
    about, 7
    ailments caused by, 7–10
    causes of, 10–13
    fighting, 17–21
    identifying, 14–15
    toxin exposure and, 13–14
cilantro, as anti-inflammatory, 31
cinnamon, as anti-inflammatory, 31
citrus fruits, as anti-inflammatory, 27
coconut
    as anti-inflammatory, 26
    coconut (or almond) milk tea, 34
    coconut oil and pineapple juice vinaigrette, 61
collard greens, as anti-inflammatory, 29
Collard Rolls, Tempeh Reuben, 95
colon cancer, 22, 27
Cookies, Trail Mix, 108–109
cooking oils, 19
coriander seeds, as anti-inflammatory, 31
corticosteroids (steroids), 17, 18
cortisol, 5, 7, 13, 18
cortisone, 18

COX enzymes
    berries/fruits and, 26, 27
    dietary fats and, 11, 19, 20
    herbs/spices and, 31, 32
    NSAIDs and, 17
cranberries, as anti-inflammatory, 26
C-reactive protein (CRP), 4, 11, 12, 15, 25
Creamy Broccoli and Cauliflower Soup, 68
Creole-Style Sweet Potato Breakfast Skillet, 45
Crohn's disease, kiwifruit and, 27
CRP (C-reactive protein), 4, 11, 12, 15, 25
cruciferous vegetables, as anti-inflammatory, 29
Crumble, Raw Stone Fruit, 111
cucumbers, as anti-inflammatory, 29
curcumin, 20, 31, 34
curry
    Black Bean and Pumpkin, 97
    curry powder, as anti-inflammatory, 31
    Sesame Dressing, Curried, Eat-the-Rainbow Salad with, 62
    sweet potato fries, curried, 91
    Tofu and Vegetable Kabobs, Curried, 98–99
Cutlets, Nut-Crusted Tofu, with Cashew Gravy, 100–101
cytokines
    about, 3–4
    aging and, 12
    antihistamines and, 17
    cancer and, 8
    C-reactive protein (CRP) and, 4
    diet and, 11
    fruits and, 27, 28
    parsley and, 31
    phytochemicals and, 20
    sleep deprivation and, 13

D

dairy products, 11, 21, 23, 32
Date Caramel Sauce, Seared Pineapple with, 109
dehydroepiandrosterone (DHEA), 12, 13
desserts. *See* sweet treats
DHA (omega-3 fat), the brain and, 18
DHEA (dehydroepiandrosterone), 12, 13
diabetes, 8, 18, 21
diet
    chronic inflammation and, 10–12
    plant foods and, 21–23
    Reinagel, Monica, and, 23
    Sears, Andrew, and, 23
    Sears, Barry, and, 15
    Western, 19

Dill-Garlic Sandwich Pickles, Refrigerator, 49
dip recipes, 50
dressing(s)
    Curried Sesame, Eat-the-Rainbow Salad
        with, 62
    lime and toasted sesame oil, 56
    Raspberry Chia-Poppy Seed, Berrylicious
        Spinach Salad with, 58
    for slaws, 54, 55
    vinaigrettes, 59, 61
Dried Fruit, Cherry-Almond Chia Pudding
    with, 105

E

Eat-the-Rainbow Salad with Curried Sesame
    Dressing, 62
edamame, as anti-inflammatory, 30
eggplants, inflammation and, 28
eggs, plant-based foods vs., 32
eicosanoids, 3, 4, 5, 8, 13
eicosapentaenoic acid (EPA), 15
EPA (eicosapentaenoic acid), 15
Escarole, White Beans with, 82
essential fatty acids/fats, 2, 3, 15, 19, 22
exercise, 12–13, 14, 15

F

farmed animals/fish, 19, 22
fat-free raspberry dressing, 58
fats (dietary), 10–11, 20, 23, 27
fermented foods
    as cancer fighter, 29
    as healthy, 21
    Pickles, Sandwich, Refrigerator Garlic-
        Dill, 49
    pickles, spicy, 49
    Sauerkraut, 48
Festive Wild Rice, 78
fish, in diet, 19, 21, 22
fish oil, 18, 22
flavonoids, 20, 30, 31
flaxseeds
    as anti-inflammatory, 25
    as high protein, 21
    omega-3s and, 19, 21, 22, 25
foods' rating system, 23
free radicals, 4–5, 8, 13, 26
Fried "Rice," Cauliflower, with Pineapple
    and Cashews, 77
fries, curried sweet potato, 91
Fries, Spicy Sweet Potato, 91
fruits. See also specific types of
    emphasizing in recipes, 32
    phytochemicals in, 20
    protein in, 21
    vs. processed foods, 21

G

garlic, as anti-inflammatory, 28
Garlic-Dill Sandwich Pickles, Refrigerator, 49
Gazpacho, Jicama, 67
ginger, as anti-inflammatory, 32
glycemic index, 23
Go Green Tea Smoothie, 37
goji berries, inflammation and, 27, 28
Gold Beet "Rice," Mexican-Style, 76
Golden Milk Tea, 34
grains. See also specific types of
    Ancient Grains, Mushroom, and Asparagus
        Medley, 75
    protein in, 21
    in Western diet, 19
gravy
    Cashew, Nut-Crusted Tofu Cutlets with,
        100–101
    mushroom-cashew, 51
    Savory Cashew, 51
Greek-style yogurt tip, 65
Green and Yellow Beans Amandine, 83
green onions and chile, paleo grits with, 42
green tea, as anti-inflammatory, 30
Green Tea Smoothie, Go, 37
greens
    Island Fruit Salad on, 61
    paleo grits with, 42
    in smoothie, 37
Grits, Paleo, 42
    with green onions and chile, 42
    with greens, 42
guava fruit, as anti-inflammatory, 27

H

Hash, Red Flannel, 46
Healthy Aging (Weil), 23
heart disease
    berries and, 26, 27
    chronic inflammation and, 8
    fish oil and, 22
    homocysteine and, 23
    hormone replacement therapy and, 12
hemp seed oil, as anti-inflammatory, 25
herbs/spices. See also specific types of
    as anti-inflammatory, 31–32
    herb-almond aioli, 52
    Mediterranean Roasted Vegetables
        with, 88–89
    phytochemicals in, 20
histamine, 3, 17

homocysteine, 23
hormone replacement therapy, chronic
    inflammation and, 12
Hot Chocolate Cake, Mexican, with Cacao
    Nibs and Nuts, 112
hydrogen peroxide, 4–5

I

ibuprofen, 2, 14, 17
immune system
    acute systemic infections and, 1
    aging and, 9
    allergies and, 2
    cortisol and, 7, 13
    fish oil and, 22
    free radicals and, 5
    garlic and, 28
    inflammation as defense for, 1, 2
    NSAIDs and, 14
    rutabaga and, 29
    smoking and, 14
    toxins and, 13
Indian-Style Tofu Scramble, 43
infections
    antioxidants and, 5
    C-reactive protein (CRP) and, 4
    herbs/spices and, 31, 32
    inflammation as response to, 1–2
    sleep deprivation and, 13
    tropical fruits and, 27
inflammaging, 9, 10
inflammation. See also specific types of
    about, 1–2
    active fighters and, 4–5
    preparatory substances and, 3–4
    reversing, 5
    Sears, Barry, and, 5, 15
    testing for, 15
    what happens during, 2–4
injuries
    chronic inflammation and, 10, 15
    free radicals and, 13
    healing substances and, 3–5, 7
    inflammation as response to, 1–2
    pineapple and, 27
insulin
    Alzheimer's disease and, 8
    body fat and, 12
    cortisol and, 7
    diabetes and, 8
    exercise and, 13
    Greek-style yogurt and, 65
    processed foods and, 21
Island Fruit Salad on Greens, 61

J

jicama, as anti-inflammatory, 29
Jicama Gazpacho, 67

K

Kabobs, Curried Tofu and Vegetable, 98–99
kale
    as anti-inflammatory, 29
    Pancakes, Shredded Vegetable and, 85
    Slaw, Omega, 55
    Stew, Roasted Winter Squash, Lentil and, 73
kidneys, rhubarb and, 28
kiwifruit, as anti-inflammatory, 27

L

latex allergy, 27
leeks, as anti-inflammatory, 28
legumes, in diet, 19, 21. *See also* specific types of legumes
lemons, as anti-inflammatory, 27
Lentil, Kale, and Roasted Winter Squash Stew, 73
lentil and rice recipe, Middle Eastern, 80–81
leukocytes, 4–5, 27
lifestyle, chronic inflammation and, 10–13, 18
lime and toasted sesame oil dressing, 56
limes, as anti-inflammatory, 27
lung cancer, citrus fruits and, 27

M

macadamia oil, as anti-inflammatory, 26
Mac-n-Cheese Cauliflower Casserole, 101
macrophages, 4, 5, 9, 30
macular degeneration, 10
main dishes
    Black Bean and Pumpkin Curry, 97
    Broccoli Rabe and White Beans with Zucchini Noodles, 102
    Mac-n-Cheese Cauliflower Casserole, 101
    Spaghetti Squash with Roasted Red Pepper Sauce, 96–97
    Tempeh Reuben Collard Rolls, 95
    Tofu and Vegetable Kabobs, Curried, 98–99
    Tofu Cutlets, Nut-Crusted, with Cashew Gravy, 100–101
    Walnut-Meat Soft Tacos, 94
maple mashed squash, 90
Maple-Glazed Squash, 90
mashed squash, maple, 90

Mayan Black Beans, 81
Mayo, Chipotle-Almond, 52
meat, 11–12, 21, 23, 32
Mediterranean Roasted Vegetables with Herb-Almond Aioli, 88–89
Medley, Squash and Cherry Tomato, 86
melanoma/skin cancer, anti-inflammatories and, 27, 31
Melon Sorbet, Minty, 104
Mexican dishes/recipes
    Mexicali Veggie Chili, 70–71
    Mexican Hot Chocolate Cake with Cacao Nibs and Nuts, 112
    Mexican-Style Gold Beet "Rice," 76
microalgae, as omega-3 source, 22
Middle Eastern lentil and rice recipe, 80–81
milk smoothie, chocolate, 36
Milk Tea, Golden, 34
Minty Melon Sorbet, 104
Miso Vegetable Soup, 64
Mujadara, 80–81
mushroom(s)
    as anti-inflammatory, 30
    Asparagus, and Ancient Grains Medley, 75
    -cashew gravy, 51
mustard greens, as anti-inflammatory, 29

N

nacho cheese sauce, spicy, 50
Napa Cabbage, Shredded, and Vegetable Salad, 56
nectarines (or peaches) in salad, 59
Neu5Gc (N-glycolyneuraminic acid), 11–12
neutrophils, 4, 5
N-glycolyneuraminic acid (Neu5Gc), 11–12
nightshade vegetables, 20, 28
no-bake fruit crumble, 111
no-cook overnight oats, 40
nonsteroidal anti-inflammatory drugs (NSAIDs), 2, 14, 17, 18, 26
Noodles, Zucchini, Broccoli Rabe and White Beans with, 102
NSAIDs (nonsteroidal anti-inflammatory drugs), 2, 14, 17, 18, 26
Nutrasource Diagnostics, 15
nut(s). *See also* specific types of nuts
    Cacao Nibs and Nuts, Mexican Hot Chocolate Cake with, 112
    essential fatty acids and, 19
    as inflammatory, 26
    Nut-Crusted Tofu Cutlets with Cashew Gravy, 100–101

Nutty Chocolate Smoothie, 36
    protein in, 21
    Vanilla-Nut Whipped Topping, 114
    in Western diet, 19

O

oat(s)
    no-cook overnight, 40
    Pancakes, Blender, 41
    Porridge, Steel-Cut, 40
obesity, 9, 12
okra, inflammation and, 28
olives, as anti-inflammatory, 30
Olives, Squash and Cherry Tomato Medley with, 86
Omega Kale Slaw, 55
omega-3s/omega-6s
    alcohol/caffeine and, 20
    Alzheimer's disease and, 8
    diet and, 11
    as essential, 2–3
    fatty fish and, 21
    fish oil and, 22
    nuts and seeds and, 21, 25
    protectins and, 5
    in recipes, 35, 55
    resolvins and, 5
    right balance of, 18–19
    Sears, Barry, and, 15
    turnip greens and, 29
onions, as anti-inflammatory, 28
oranges, as anti-inflammatory, 27
oregano, as anti-inflammatory, 31
overnight oats, no-cook, 40

P

Paleo Grits, 42
    with green onions and chile, 42
    with greens, 42
Pancakes, Blender Oat, 41
Pancakes, Shredded Vegetable and Kale, 85
papaya, as anti-inflammatory, 27
paprika, inflammation and, 28
Parfaits, Tropical Fruit, 107
Parkinson's disease, 31
parsley, as anti-inflammatory, 31
peaches (or nectarines) in salad, 59
Pecan, Pomegranate, and Stone Fruit Salad, 59
peppermint, as anti-inflammatory, 31
phytochemicals, 20, 23, 26, 27
Pickles, Sandwich, Refrigerator Garlic-Dill, 49
pickles, spicy, 49

pineapple
  as anti-inflammatory, 27
  *and Cashews, Cauliflower Fried "Rice"
    with*, 77
    pineapple juice and coconut oil
      vinaigrette, 61
  Seared, with Date Caramel Sauce, 109
plant-based foods/recipes, 22, 32
polyphenols, 20, 26
Pomegranate, Stone Fruit, and Pecan Salad,
  59
pomegranate vinaigrette, 59
*Poppy Seed-Raspberry Chia Dressing,
  Berrylicious Spinach Salad with*, 58
Porridge, Steel-Cut Oats, 40
potatoes, inflammation and, 28
prednisone, 18
preparatory substances, 3–4
probiotics, 21
processed (refined) foods, 10–12, 19, 21, 30
pro-inflammatory reaction
  animal products and, 11
  eicosanoids and, 3, 4, 8
  myokines and, 13
  symptoms, 2
  weight and, 12, 21
prostaglandins, 20, 27
prostate cancer, walnuts to fight against,
  25
protectins, 5
*Pudding, Cherry-Almond Chia, with Dried
  Fruit*, 105
pumpkin(s)
  as anti-inflammatory, 29
  -Chipotle Soup, Smoky, 69
  Curry, Black Bean and, 97

R
*Rainbow Salad, Eat-the-, with Curried
  Sesame Dressing*, 62
raspberries, as anti-inflammatory, 26
*Raspberry Chia-Poppy Seed Dressing,
  Berrylicious Spinach Salad with*, 58
rating system for foods, 23
Raw Stone Fruit Crumble, 111
Red Flannel Hash, 46
*Red Pepper Sauce, Roasted, Spaghetti Squash
  with*, 96–97
refined (processed) foods, 10–12, 19, 20,
  21, 30
Refrigerator Garlic-Dill Sandwich Pickles, 49
Reinagel, Monica, 23
resolvins, 5
resveratrol, 20

Reuben Collard Rolls, Tempeh, 95
rhubarb, as anti-inflammatory, 28
Rhubarb and Strawberries, Stewed, 110
rice
  *Cauliflower Fried "Rice," with Pineapple
    and Cashews*, 77
  Festive Wild, 78
  and lentil recipe, Middle Eastern, 80–81
  Mexican-Style Gold Beet "Rice," 76
roasted dishes/recipes
  Brussels Sprouts, 92
  Red Pepper Sauce, Spaghetti Squash with,
    96–97
  *Vegetables, Mediterranean, with Herb-
    Almond Aioli*, 88–89
  Winter Squash, Lentil, and Kale Stew, 73
Rolls, Tempeh Reuben Collard, 95
root vegetables, as anti-inflammatory, 29
Root Vegetables, Whipped, 87
rutabaga, as anti-inflammatory, 29

S
salad(s)
  *Berrylicious Spinach, with Raspberry
    Chia-Poppy Seed Dressing*, 58
  *Eat-the-Rainbow, with Curried Sesame
    Dressing*, 62
  Island Fruit, on Greens, 61
  Napa Cabbage and Vegetable, Shredded,
    56
  Stone Fruit, Pecan, and Pomegranate, 59
Sandwich Pickles, Refrigerator Garlic-Dill,
  49
sauce(s)
  cashew
    Cheese, 50
    cheese dip, smoky, 50
    Gravy, Savory, 51
    cheese, spicy nacho, 50
  Date Caramel, Seared Pineapple with,
    109
  *Roasted Red Pepper, Spaghetti Squash
    with*, 96–97
Sauerkraut, 48
sauerkraut, as anti-inflammatory, 29
Savory Cashew Gravy, 51
Scramble, Tofu, Indian-Style, 43
Seared Pineapple with Date Caramel Sauce,
  109
Sears, Barry, 5, 15
  The Anti-Inflammation Zone, 5
seeds. *See also* specific types of
  as anti-inflammatory, 25
  essential fatty acids and, 19

protein in, 21
  in Western diet, 19
Sesame Dressing, Curried, 62
sesame oil dressing, toasted, lime and, 56
shallots, as anti-inflammatory, 28
*Shredded Napa Cabbage and Vegetable
  Salad*, 56
Shredded Vegetable and Kale Pancakes, 85
side dishes
  Black Beans, Mayan, 81
  Brussels Sprouts, Roasted, 92
  Green and Yellow Beans Amandine, 83
  Mujadara, 80–81
  *Mushroom, Asparagus, and Ancient
    Grains Medley*, 75
  rice
    *Cauliflower Fried "Rice" with
      Pineapple and Cashews*, 77
    Festive Wild, 78
    Gold Beet "Rice," Mexican-Style, 76
  Root Vegetables, Whipped, 87
  Sauerkraut, 48
  Squash, Maple-Glazed, 90
  *Squash and Cherry Tomato Medley with
    Olives*, 86
  Sweet Potato Fries, Spicy, 91
  Vegetable, Shredded, and Kale Pancakes,
    85
  *Vegetables, Mediterranean Roasted, with
    Herb-Almond Aioli*, 88–89
  White Beans with Escarole, 82
Skillet, Breakfast, Creole-Style Sweet Potato,
  45
skin cancer/melanoma, anti-
  inflammatories and, 27, 31
Slaw, Bavarian, 54
Slaw, Omega Kale, 55
sleep deprivation, chronic inflammation
  and, 13
smoking, as toxic, 14
smoky cashew cheese dip, 50
Smoky Pumpkin-Chipotle Soup, 69
Smoothie, Berry Blast-Off, 35
Smoothie Bowl, Superfood, 38
Soft Tacos, Walnut-Meat, 94
Sorbet, Minty Melon, 104
soup(s)
  Borscht, 65
  Broccoli and Cauliflower, Creamy, 68
  Jicama Gazpacho, 67
  Miso Vegetable, 64
  Pumpkin-Chipotle, Smoky, 69
  White Bean and Swiss Chard, 72
soy foods, as anti-inflammatory, 30